Notes

Some of our topics cover:

Heart disease	Diabetes	Asthma
Heart disease risk factors	Nutrition	Chronic lung disease
Heart surgery	Exercise	Hip or knee surgery
High blood pressure	Head injury	Bowel surgery
Stroke	Home care	

Write or call toll-free for a free catalog of products and prices:

1-800-241-4925

I0123211

Use this book to learn about:

Treatment Choices:

® Order this book from :

PRITCHETT & HULL ASSOCIATES, INC.
3440 OAKCLIFF RD NE STE 126
ATLANTA GA 30340-3006
or call toll free: 800-241-4925

Published and distributed by:
Pritchett & Hull Associates, Inc.
Printed in the U.S.A.

This book is written to help you
understand kidney failure. It should not
be used to replace any of your doctor's
advice or treatment.

Where Pritchett & Hull Associates, Inc.
was aware of names of products for
which a trademark has been claimed,
such names have been printed in initial
capital letters (e.g., Jell-O).

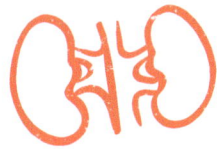

KIDNEY FAILURE

coping & feeling your best

by Anna K. Hollingsworth, MPH, RN, CHES

Dear Reader,

It has been an honor to write this book. As a nurse, I care about those with kidney failure. And as a person with kidney disease who has had a kidney removed, I have a special interest in making sure you have good education materials.

— Anna

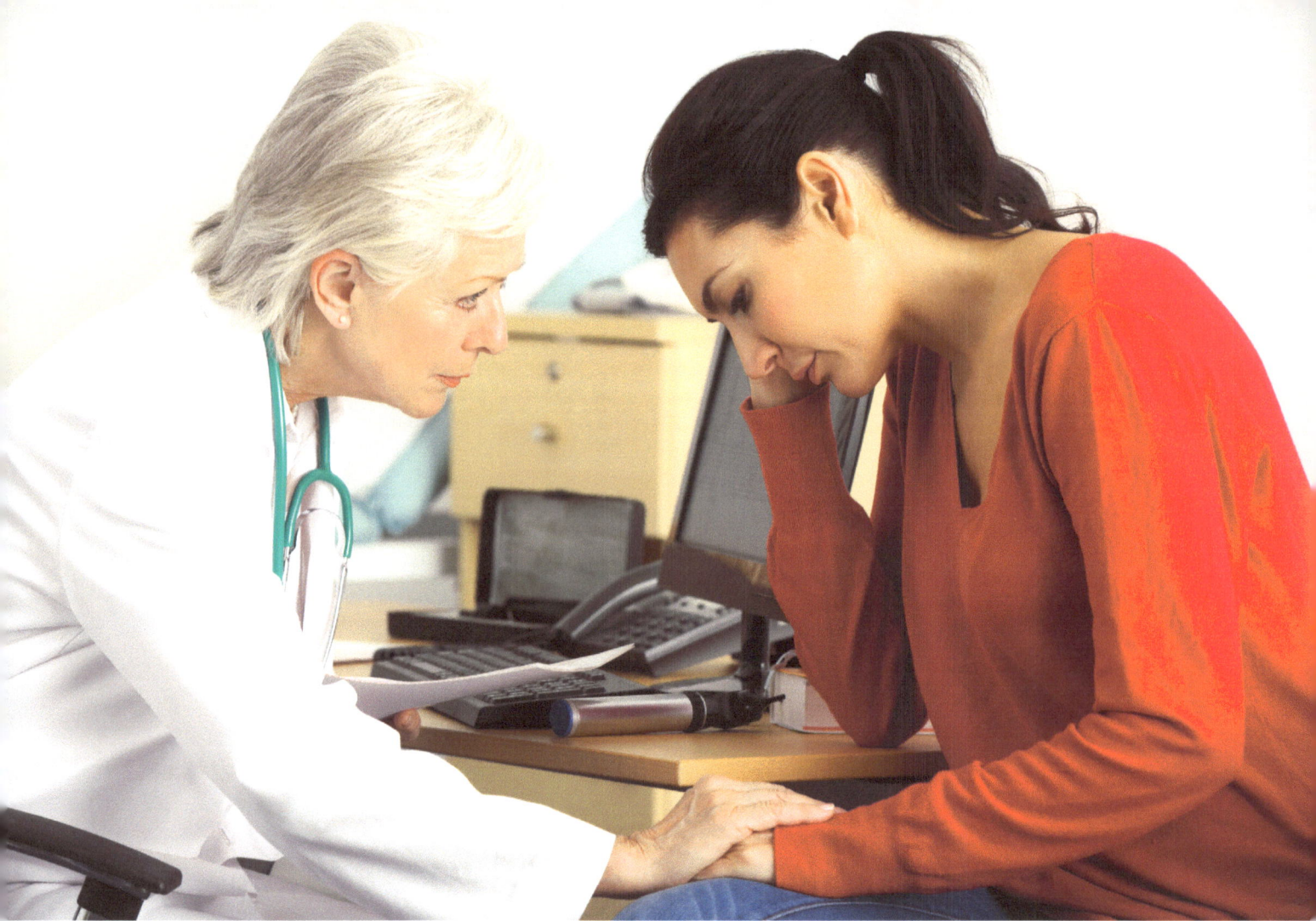

What is kidney failure?

You may feel overwhelmed when your doctor talks to you about your kidney failure. The news about your kidney failure may seem like a blur. Sometimes the waste in your blood can cause that. When your kidneys can't remove fluid, waste products (waste) and electrolytes (salt*) from your body, it is called kidney failure. Your kidneys also help control blood pressure and the making of red blood cells. When your kidneys fail, they can no longer do these jobs.

*Substances such as potassium and sodium

How did you get it?

Your kidney failure may be caused by one of these:

high blood
pressure

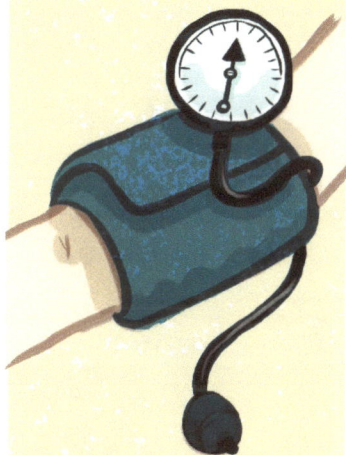

diabetes that is
not controlled

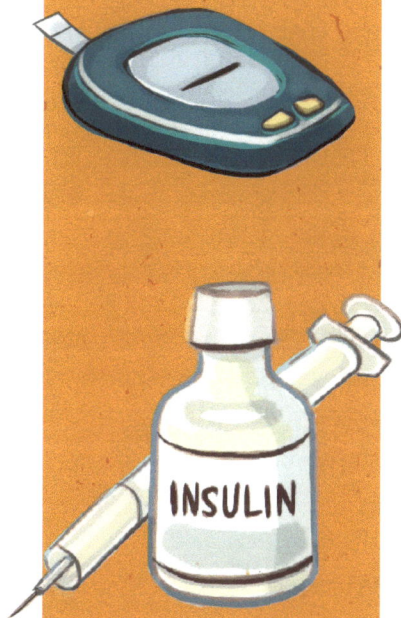

kidney infections,
kidney stones,
infected kidneys,
gout, lupus

taking some over-
the-counter drugs
for a long time

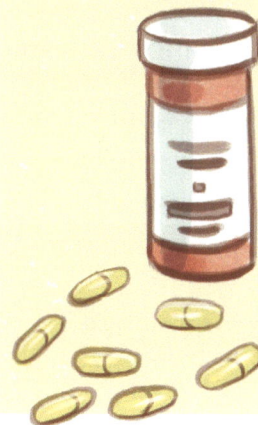

INSULIN

These are only the main causes. Ask your doctor if one of these or
something else caused your kidney failure.

Why does kidney failure make you feel so sick?

When your kidneys fail, fluid, waste and salt builds up in your body. Your blood pressure may get very high, and your body won't make enough red blood cells. All of this makes you feel sick. You may notice:

- a bad taste in your mouth, bad breath

- feeling sick to your stomach (nausea)

- puffiness around your eyes

- shortness of breath and swelling in your feet, ankles and wrists

- less urine, dark, bloody urine; and/or burning when you urinate

- urinating more often (more often at night)

- headaches

- feeling tired and run down

- skipped heartbeats

- low back pain (just below your ribs)

You will most likely "feel bad all over," but feeling like this is common before you start treatment.

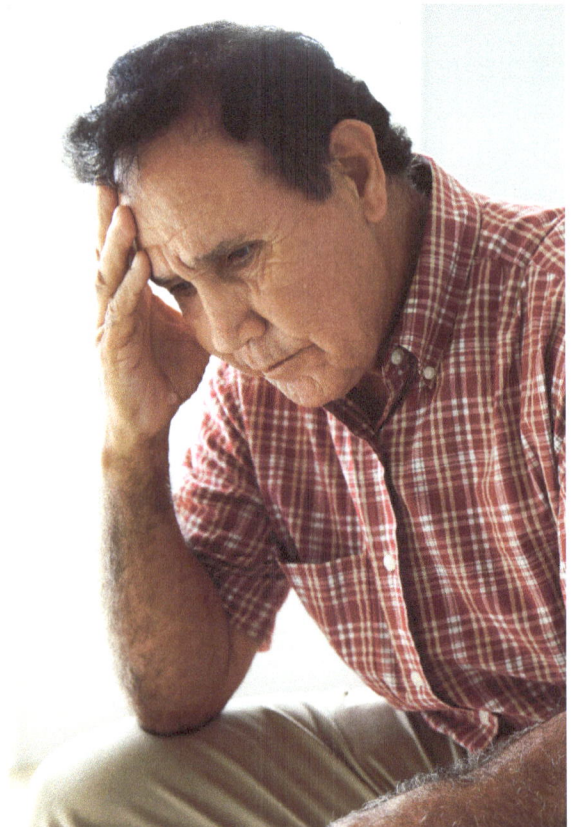

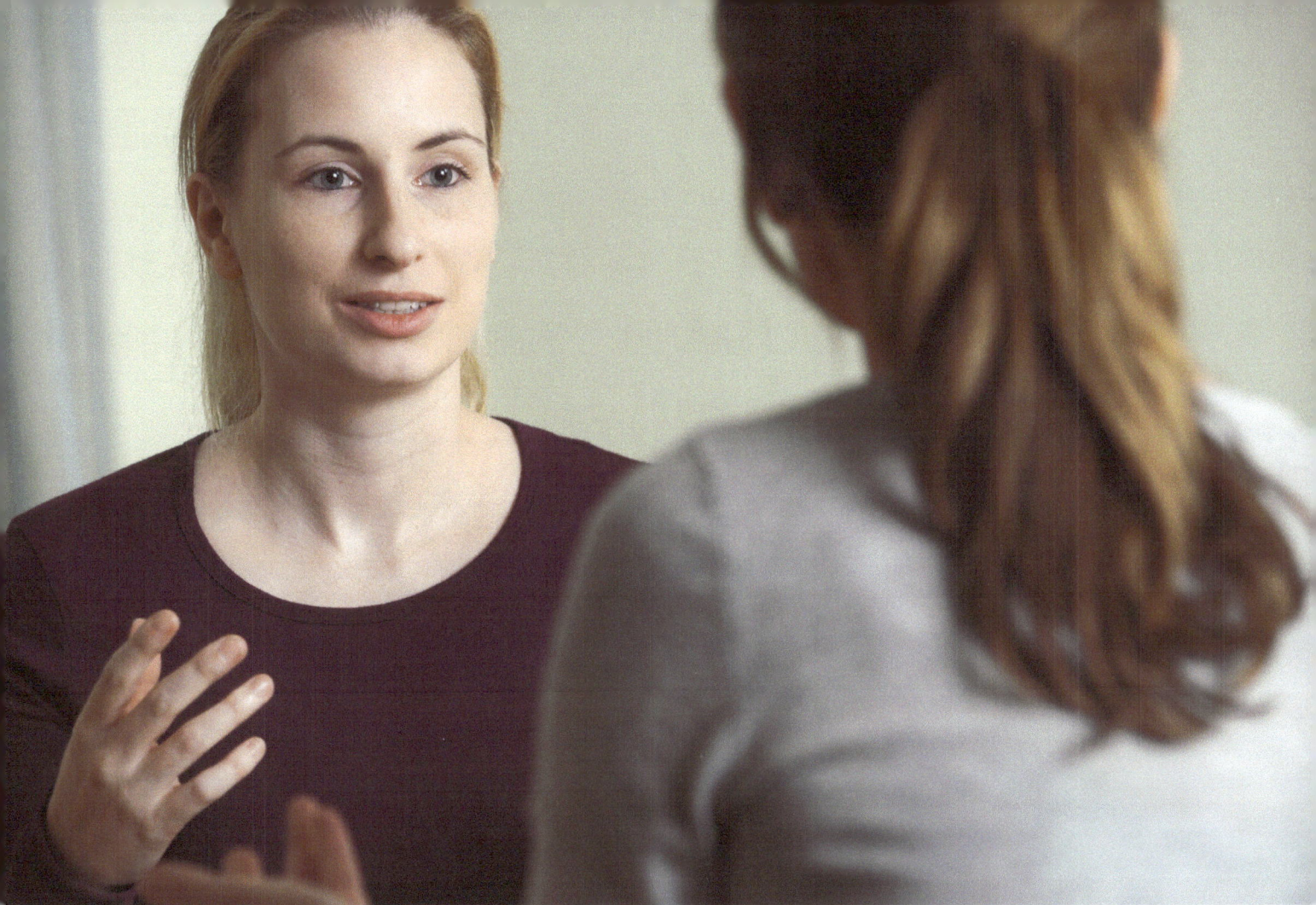

What helps you feel better?

You will begin to feel better when you can get rid of the extra fluid, waste and salt in your body. The next pages will tell you how to do this.

Your failed kidneys can't be fixed, but you can be treated. Treatment for kidney failure will have to be done for the rest of your life.

Kidney failure is hard on you, and it's normal to be scared. It affects every aspect of your life. You may also feel angry, sad and have many other feelings as you learn to cope with the changes in your life. All of this may seem like too much to think about. When the first shock is over and you begin to work out a new routine for your life, these feelings will not be as strong. Family and friends will also learn how they can support you so that all of you can get on with your lives.

What about the long haul?

Treatment for kidney failure has 3 main parts.
You will do these for the rest of your life:

clean (filter) your blood	take medicine	eat a special diet and limit fluids

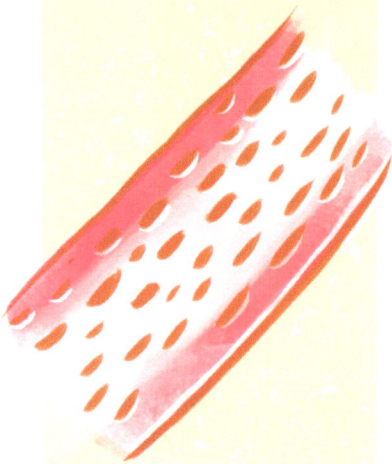

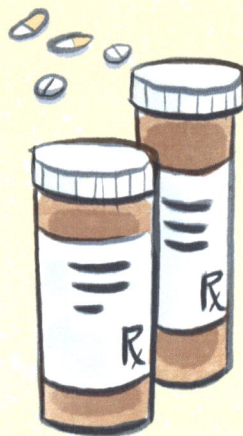

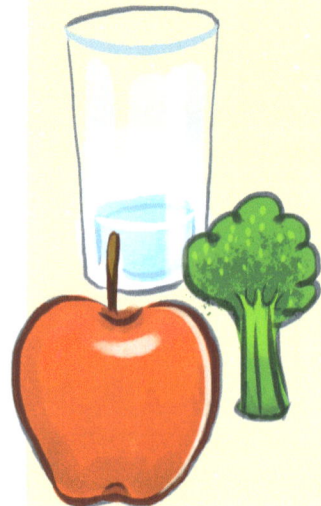

Your doctor will choose the diet and medicines that are best for you and will guide you in your choice of treatment. The choice may be one of these:

- dialysis

- kidney transplant

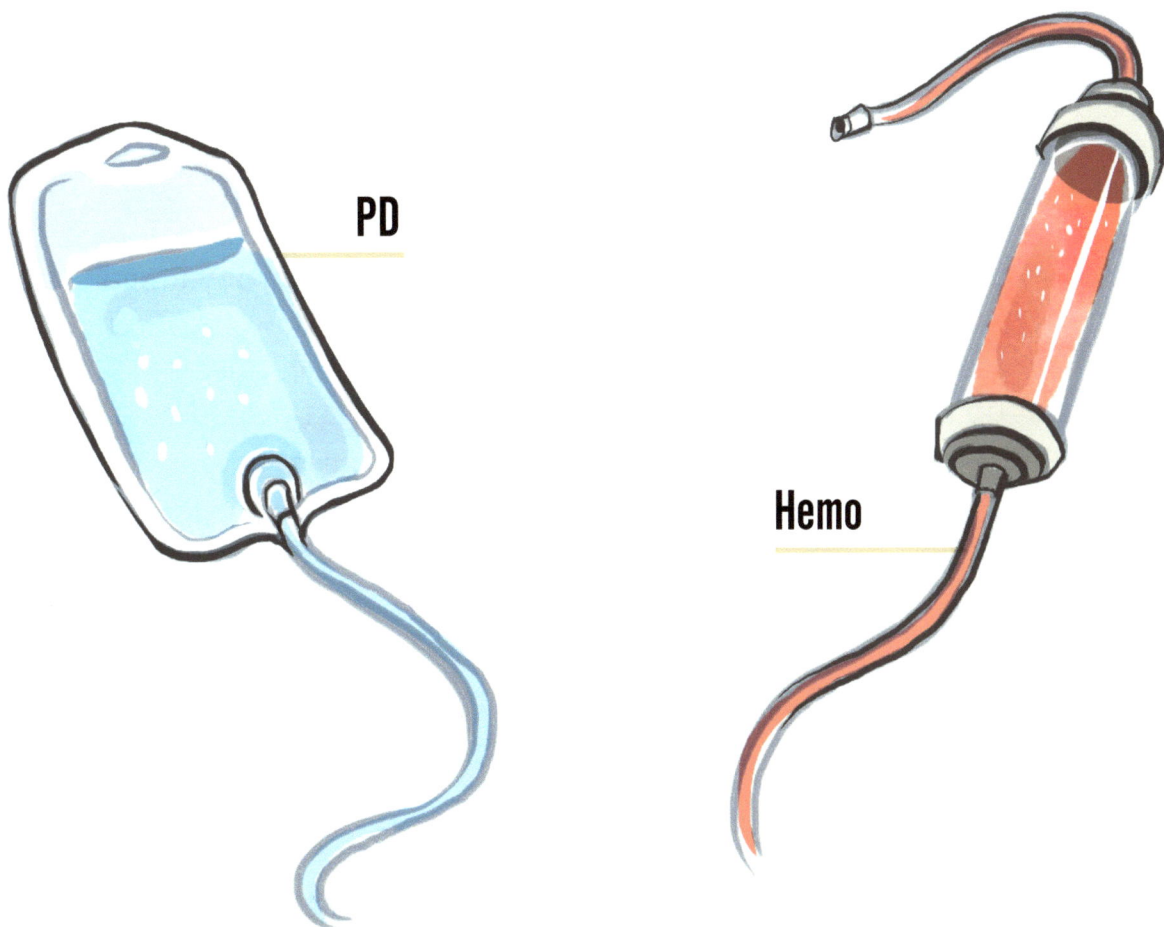

PD

Hemo

Dialysis

Dialysis cleans your blood. There are two kinds: peritoneal dialysis **(PD)** and hemodialysis **(hemo)**. With PD, your blood stays in the body to be cleaned. With hemo, your blood is cleaned outside the body in an artificial kidney.

There is a lot to know about both PD and hemo. When you know which dialysis you will use, read these pages to find out more:

- pages 16 – 27 for more on PD

- pages 28 – 41 for more on hemo

Kidney transplant

Another choice for you might be a kidney transplant. This means placing a kidney from someone else inside your body. With a new kidney, you would no longer have to have dialysis, but you would still have to take special care of yourself.

You may have a family member who can donate a kidney, or you may be put on a waiting list until a kidney that matches you can be found. Because there aren't enough kidneys to go around, strict rules have been set up to decide who will get one. You may not be placed on a waiting list if you:

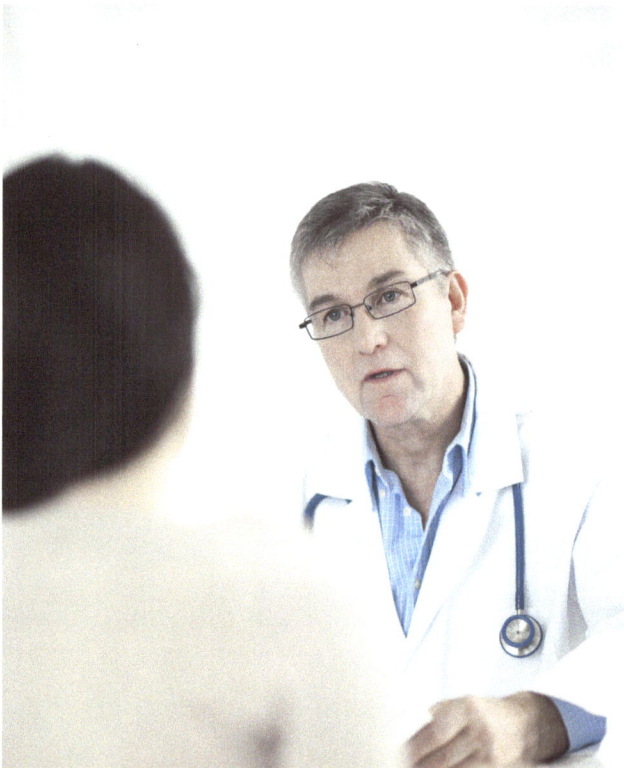

- have cancer, AIDS or certain heart diseases

- have a drug or alcohol problem

- do not stick to your diet, medicines and other treatment

If you are put on a kidney waiting list, some tests will be done to make sure that the new kidney is a good match for you.

Having a kidney transplant will let you eat a more normal diet than if you are on dialysis. But you will still have to limit salt and take many medicines. You will also need to visit your doctor often for blood and urine tests.

Sometimes a person's body may try to reject the new kidney. This can start months, or even years, after the transplant. For some, another kidney may be a choice. Others may have to go back on dialysis.

If you can't think straight now

It is normal not to be able to think well right now. Chances are your mind is not clear due to the waste in your blood and the shock of finding out that you have a serious illness.

The good news is that you do not have to make up your mind about long-term treatment right away. You are already getting short-term treatment, and very soon you will be able to think more clearly. Right now you need the support of family and friends. Call on them during this time, and let them know what they can do. **Make a list on page 10 to get started.**

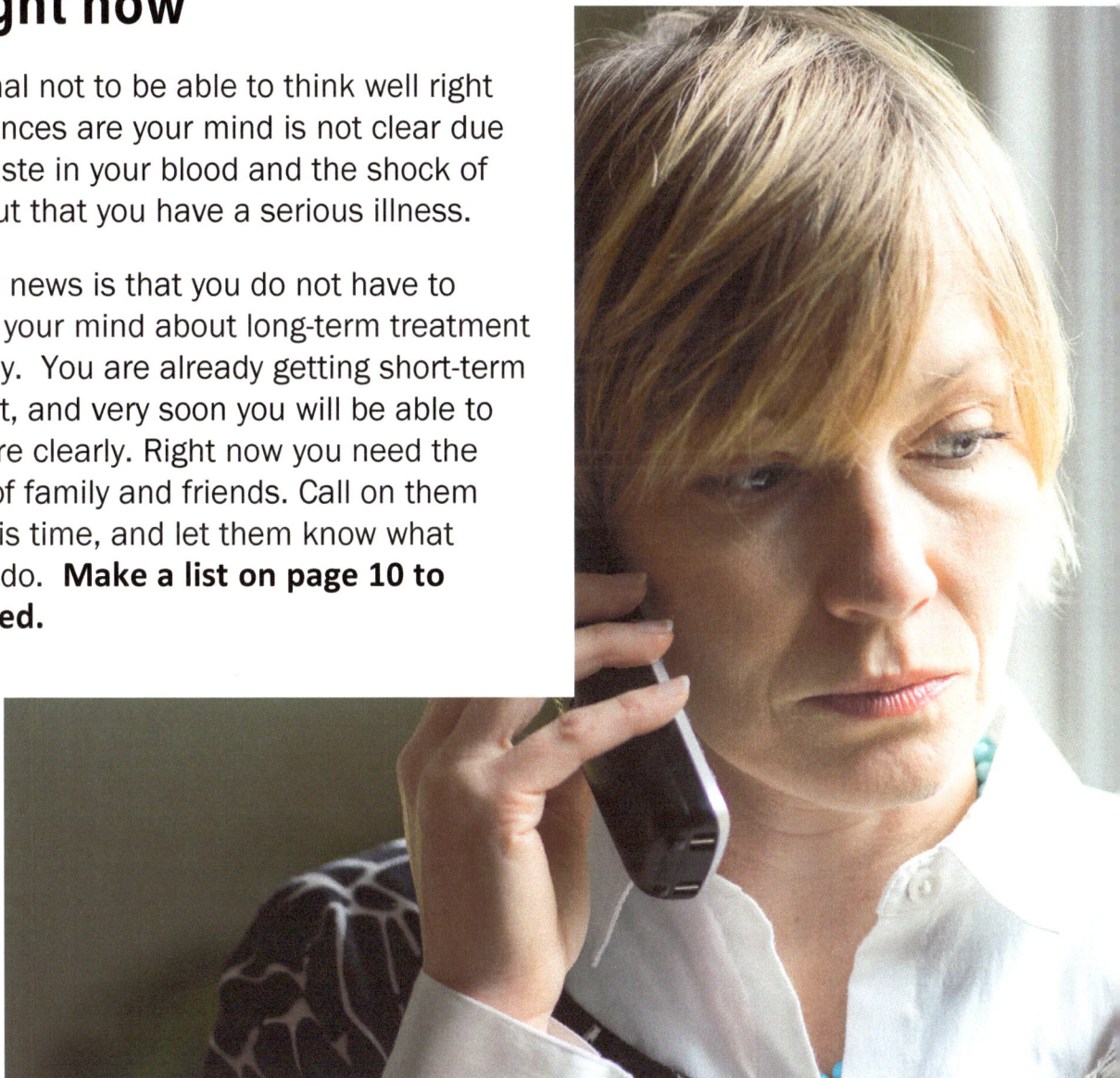

Use this space to make a list of people you can call on for support.

name	phone number	how he or she can help

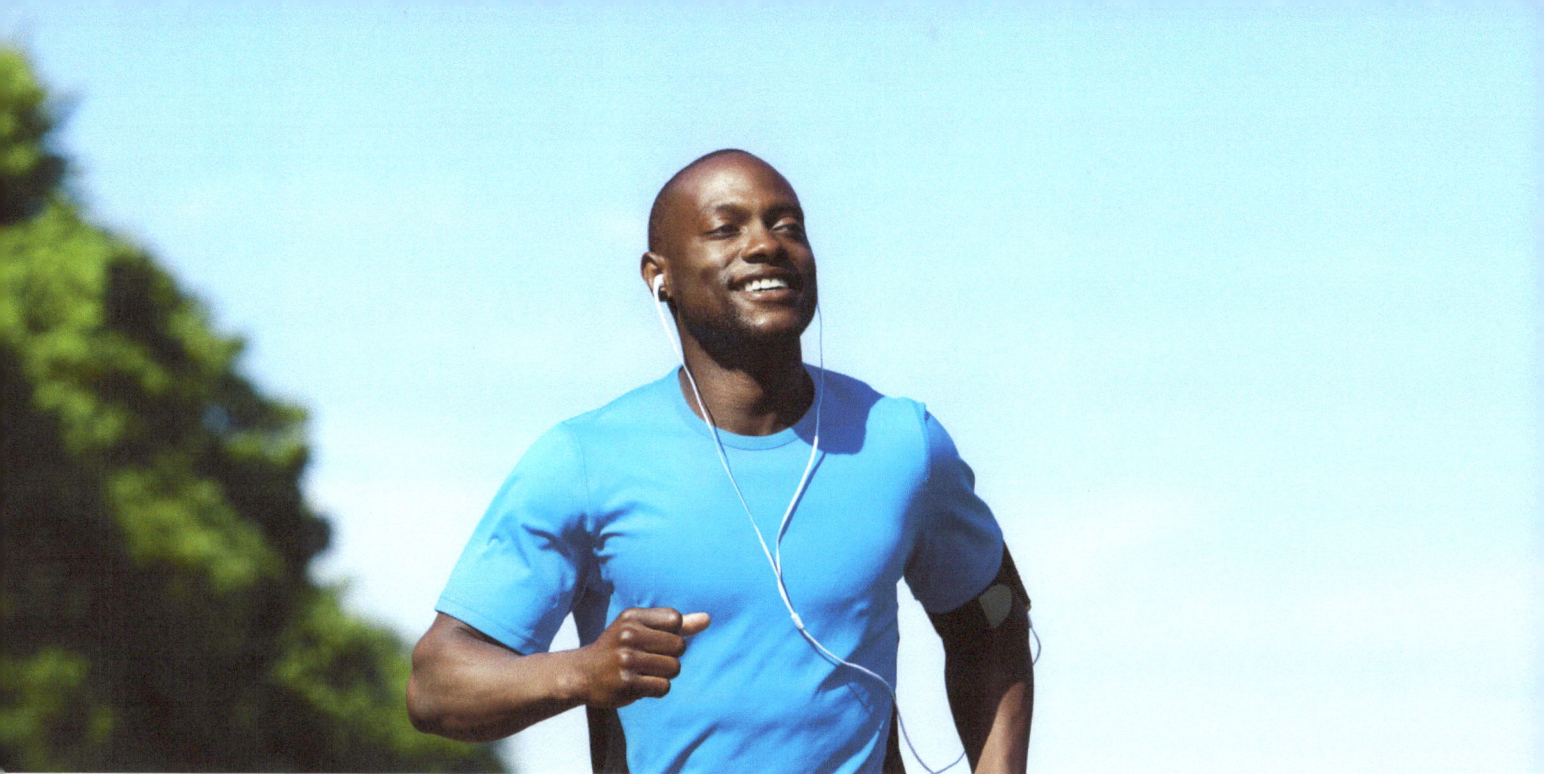

So which treatment is best?

The treatment you end up with depends on:

- your past illnesses

- how sick you are right now

- your age

- your habits or lifestyle

Your doctor will help guide you to the choice that's best for you.

It can also be your choice **not** to have treatment. Some people choose this. They may already have some other serious illness such as cancer or severe heart disease. Often these people say they feel that treatment would just prolong death, not extend life.

The no-treatment choice is a personal and serious one. If you are thinking about this, talk it over with your family, nurse and doctor. Whatever choice you make should be the right one for you.

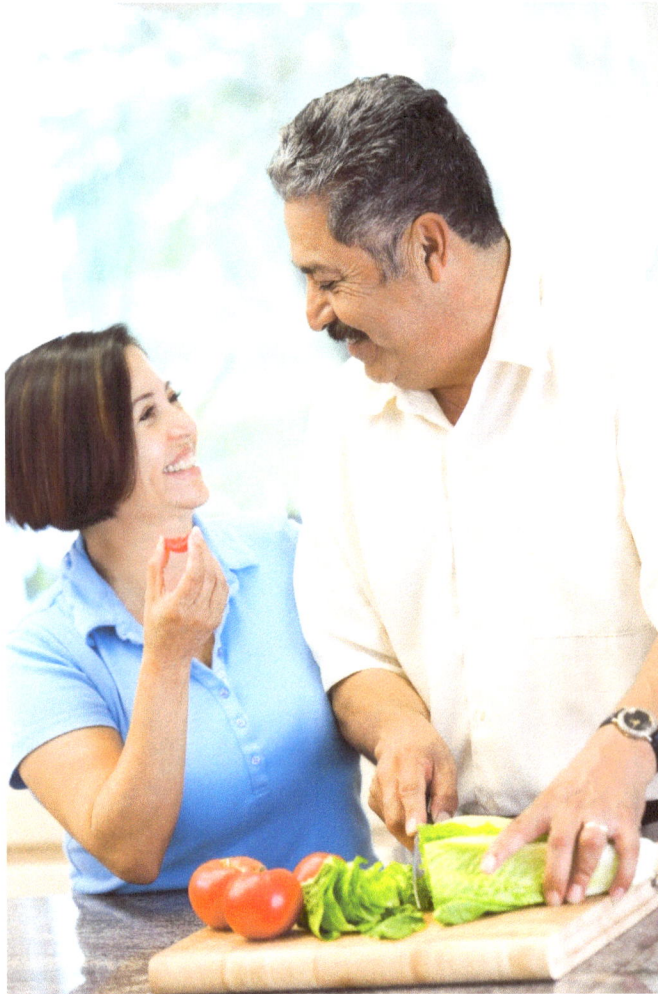

How will kidney failure change your life?

There will be many changes, but your whole life does not have to change. Each year thousands of new kidney failure patients learn to cope.

➡ diet

You must eat a special diet and learn to fix the foods you can eat. Some foods have to be measured, and others must be cooked in special ways. You will also have to limit your fluid intake. A dietitian will help you learn about your diet and how to measure fluid amounts.

➡ blood pressure check

You may need to check your blood pressure at home. This is easy to do, and you or a family member can learn how in less than an hour.

Medicine chart

For:
name_____
address_____
phone_____

Doctor:_____
address_____
phone_____

Pharmacy:
address_____
phone_____

Dialysis Clinic:
address_____
phone_____

date   weight   when to take   how much   things to watch for

© Pritchett & Hull Associates, Inc. Atlanta, GA Patients

medicine

You and a family member or friend must learn all about your medicine: what it's for, what it looks like and when and how much to take. You can use the chart on page 48 to help keep track of this.

exercise

Exercise is good for your body and mind. Make an exercise plan with your doctor, and stick to it.

weight

Learn to watch your weight. A weight gain often means you have taken in too much fluid.

identification (ID)

Wear some kind of ID at all times. There are nice bracelets or necklaces for this purpose. An ID lets others know you have kidney failure if for some reason you can't tell them yourself. (Ask your nurse how to get one.)

depression

Depression is more than just being sad for a short time. It is an illness with its own warning signs, and it can be treated. It's normal for people with kidney failure to get depressed. You and those close to you should know these signs to watch for so you can seek help when needed:

- feeling restless or slowed down

- feeling tired all the time, lack of energy

- feeling sad or blue (discouraged)

- trouble thinking, remembering, concentrating or making decisions

- losing interest in things you used to enjoy

- change in weight or appetite

- trouble sleeping or sleeping too much

- feeling guilty or worthless

- having thoughts of death or suicide*

*If you feel this way, this is a medical emergency– you need to call your doctor or 911 or go to the emergency room right away!

List adapted from Depression: A Treatable Illness (Fact Sheet) National Institute of Mental Health NIH Publication number TR-10-3561.

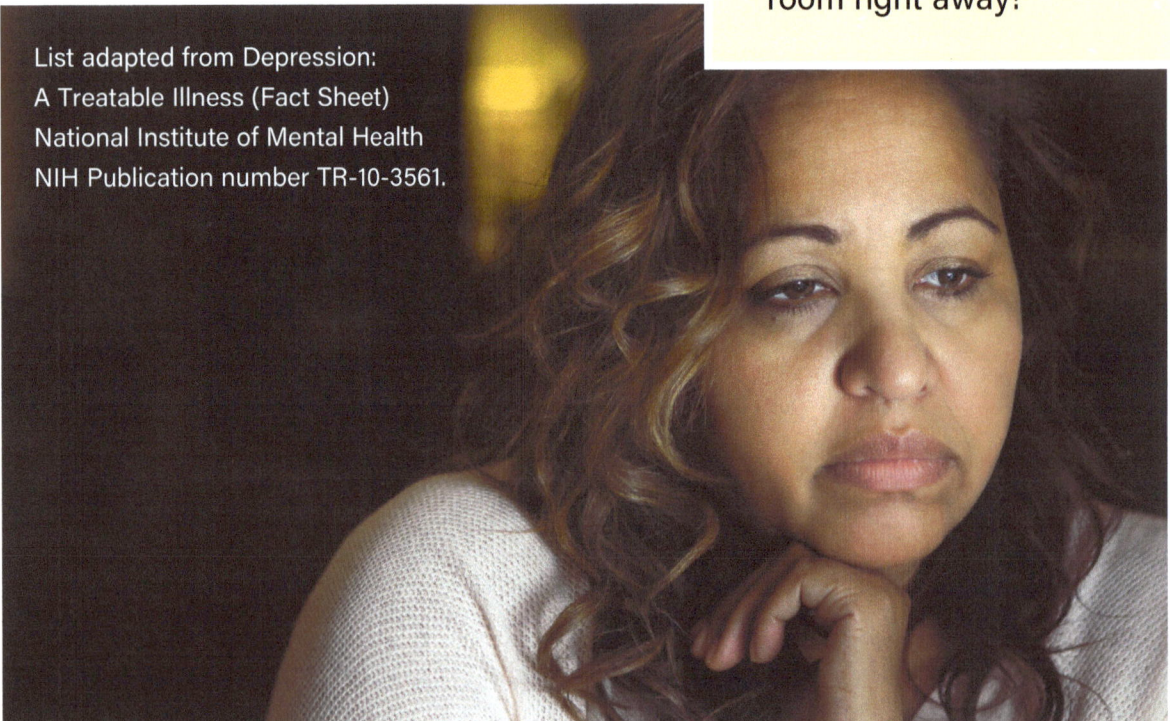

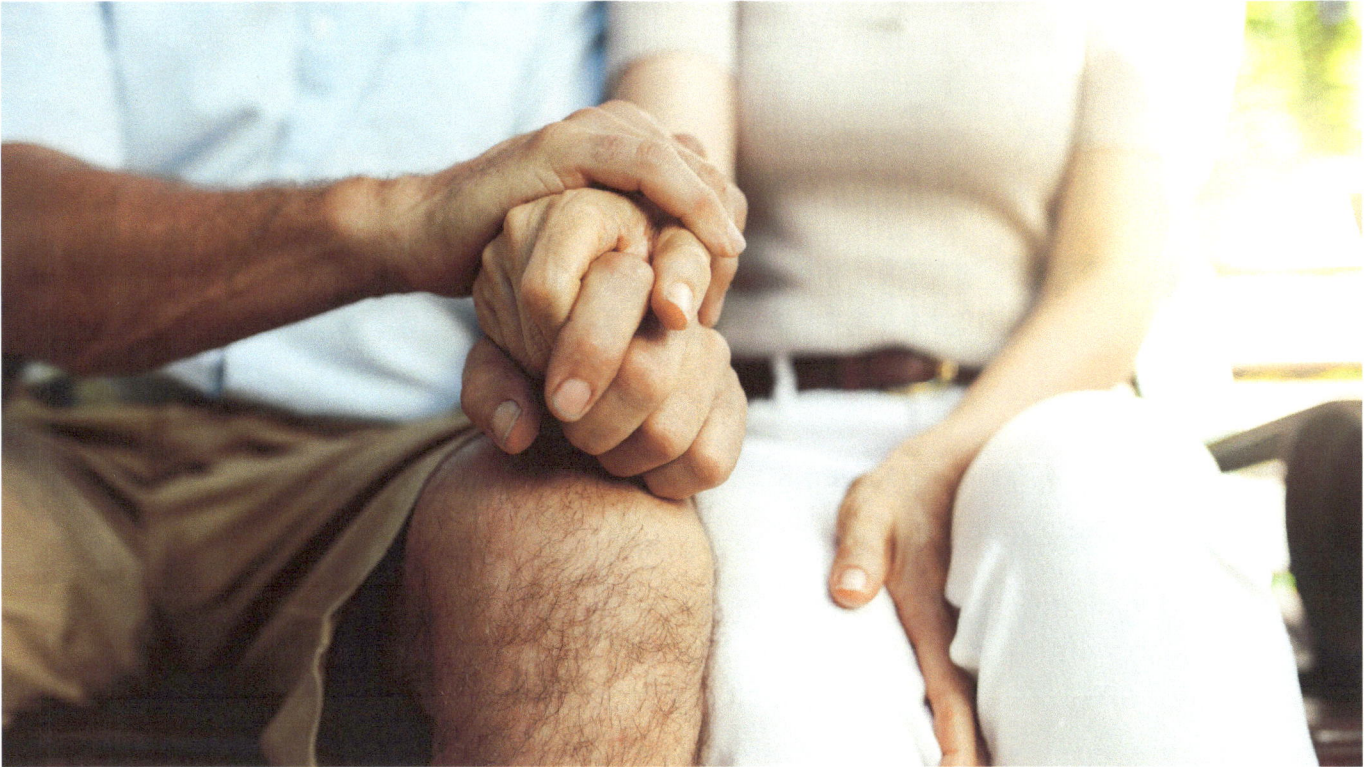

▶ going places

If you are on hemo, you will need someone to take you to and from your treatments at first. You may be able to drive yourself to your treatments later on.

▶ emotional support

You and your family need a lot of support during this time. You can talk with each other, but you each need someone else you can talk to. Social workers, nurses, doctors, church members and friends can help.

Sometimes a family gives up all outside interests to care for a loved one. This is not good. Family members need to take special care of themselves, too. They need to get plenty of rest, eat well and keep up some outside activities.

▶ sex

Both men and women may have changes in sexual desire. Some men may have trouble having an erection. You can still enjoy sex, but you and your partner may need to find new ways. Ask your doctor or nurse to talk about this with you. There are many things that can be done to help, and some resources are listed on page 46.

More about PD (Peritoneal Dialysis)

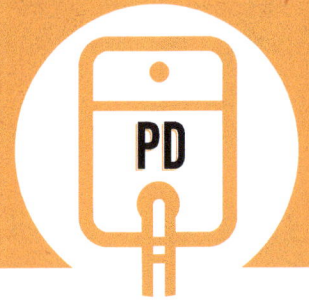

PD

PD cleans your blood by using a natural membrane already inside your belly to filter your blood.

Fluid, called dialysate, is put into your abdomen (belly). This fluid draws excess water and waste through the membrane. Then all of it (dialysate, water and waste) is drained back out of your belly.

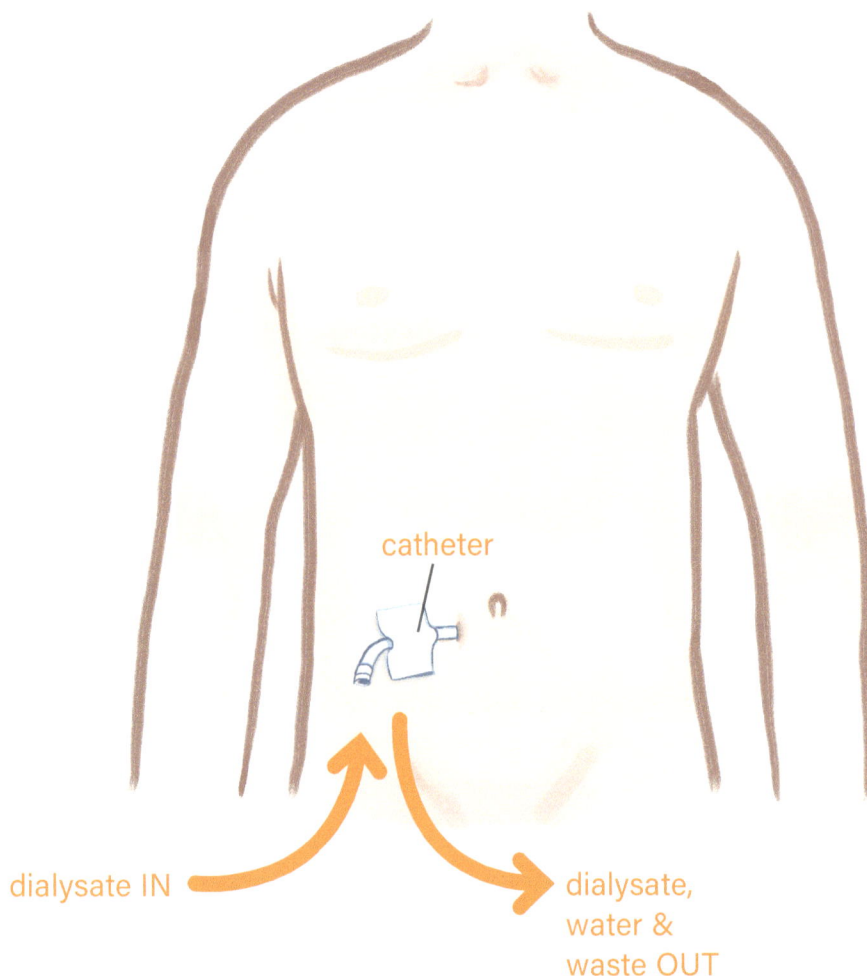

catheter

dialysate IN

dialysate, water & waste OUT

How does the fluid get inside?

The doctor puts a tube, called a PD catheter, into your belly. This is done with a short surgery or by a simple puncture. Most of the time, you do not have to be put to sleep. The tube won't leak or show through your clothes, and you will be taught how to keep it clean to avoid infection. The tube stays in place as long as you are on PD.

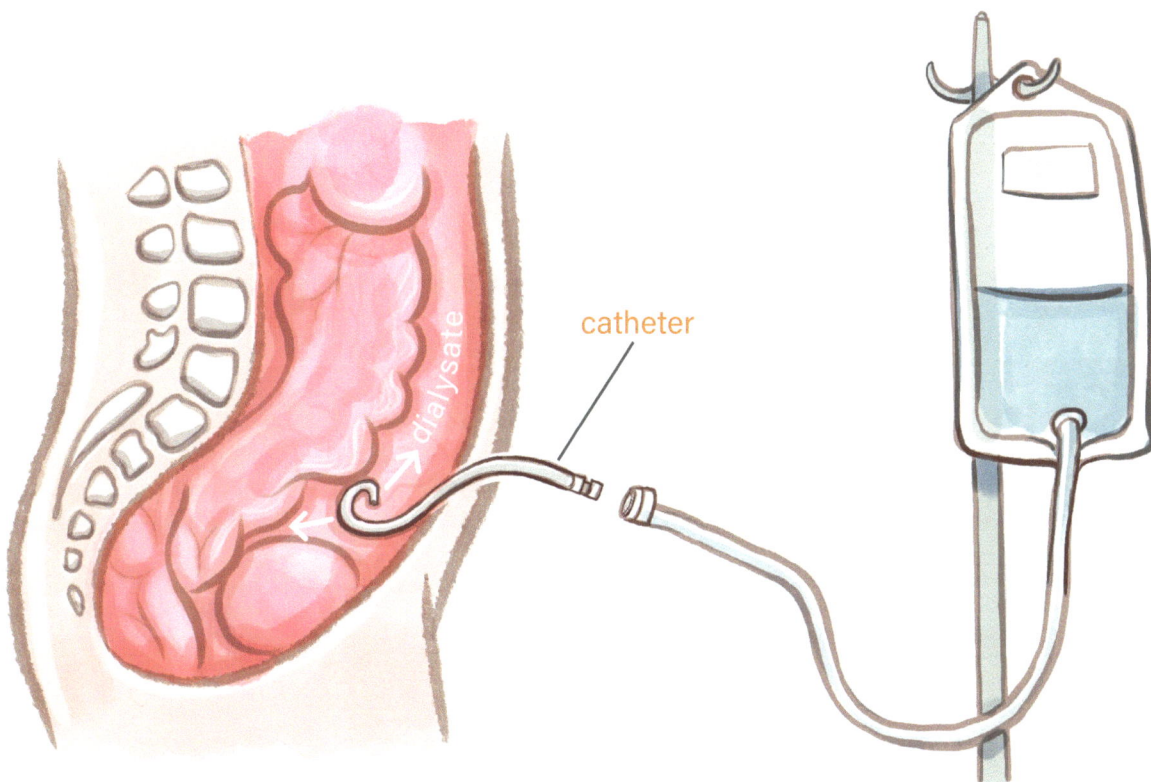

catheter

dialysate

Once your PD catheter is in place, you can begin your treatments. You may take them **overnight, or** you may do PD **throughout the day.** You and your doctor will decide which method is best for you.

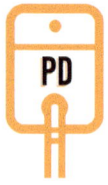

Overnight PD
(called CCPD or continuous cycling peritoneal dialysis)

For overnight PD, you use a machine which warms the fluid and lets it in and out of your belly. You will set up your machine, then hook a long tube to your PD catheter and let in the warmed dialysate.

After ¾ to 1½ hours, the dialysate is drained off and thrown away. The machine repeats this process many times during the night. If you use this type of PD, someone will teach you how to use and care for your machine.

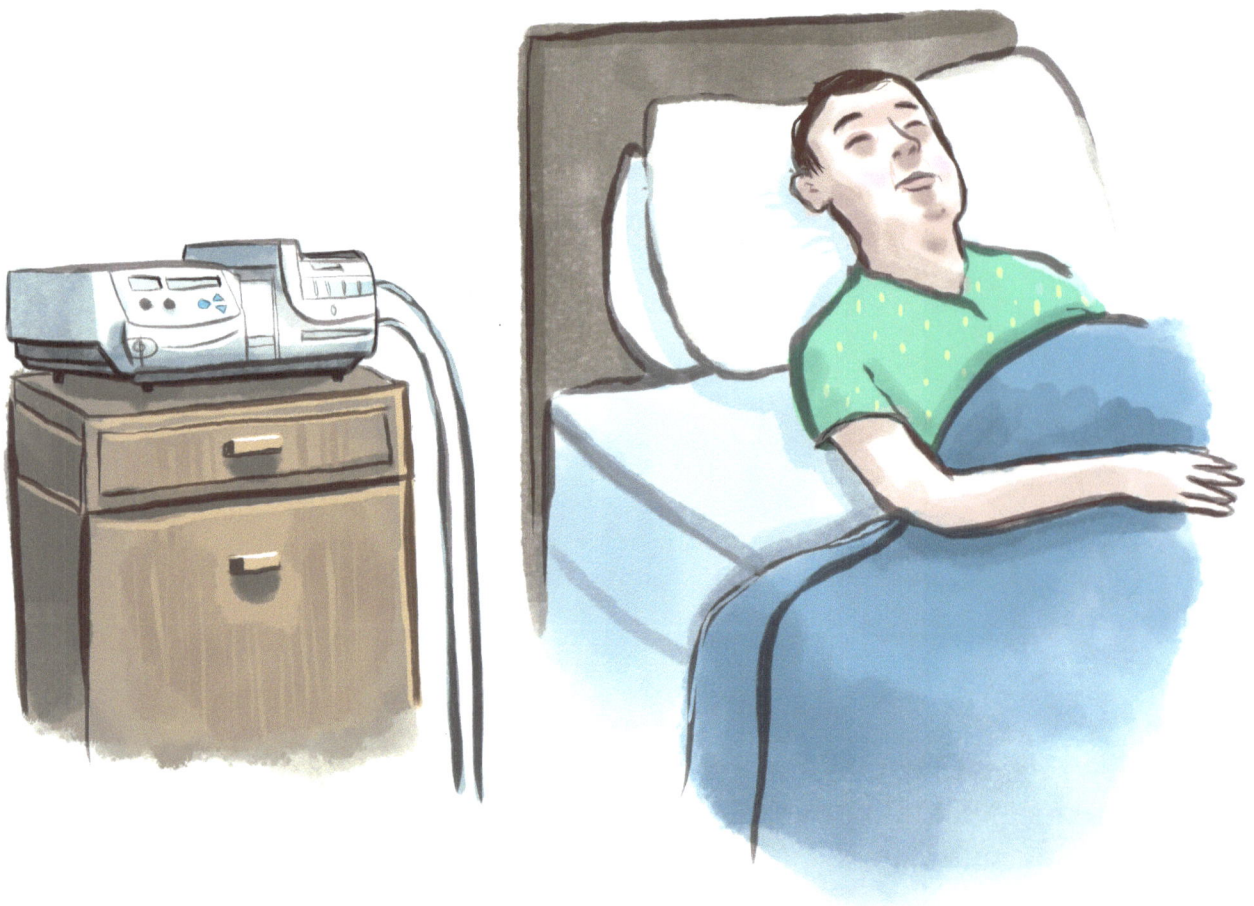

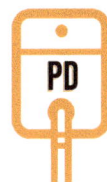

Continuous PD
(called CAPD or continuous ambulatory peritoneal dialysis)

You do this type of PD during the day and night, without a machine. For most people, it takes about a week to learn how to do it. You use a tube to hook a bag of warmed dialysate to your catheter and let the fluid drain in. Once the fluid is in, you are free to move about as you wish.

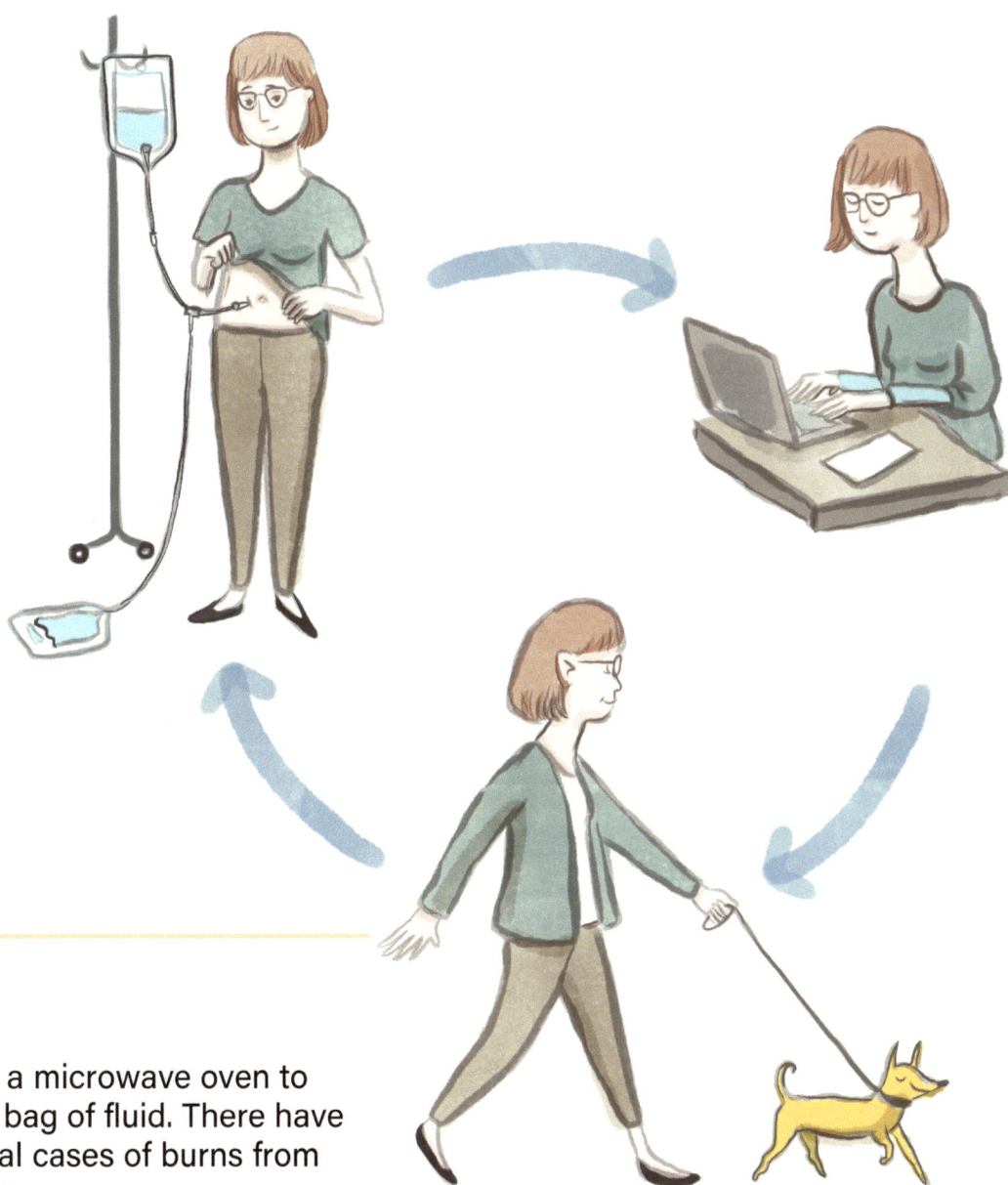

Caution

Do not use a microwave oven to warm your bag of fluid. There have been several cases of burns from overheating.

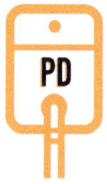

The fluid stays in for 4 to 6 hours, then is let out. To do this, you drain the dialysate, plus the extra fluid and waste products it has gathered, into an empty bag. Set the empty bag down in a clean place below your belly. Some people spread a clean towel on the floor, others use a footstool. Connect a tube from your catheter to the bag, and let the fluid drain. As soon as you finish draining, put another warmed bag of dialysate into your belly.

The whole process of draining out and putting in fluid is called an exchange and takes about 30 minutes. **You must take care to do your exchanges in a clean place and just as you have been taught. This will help prevent infection.**

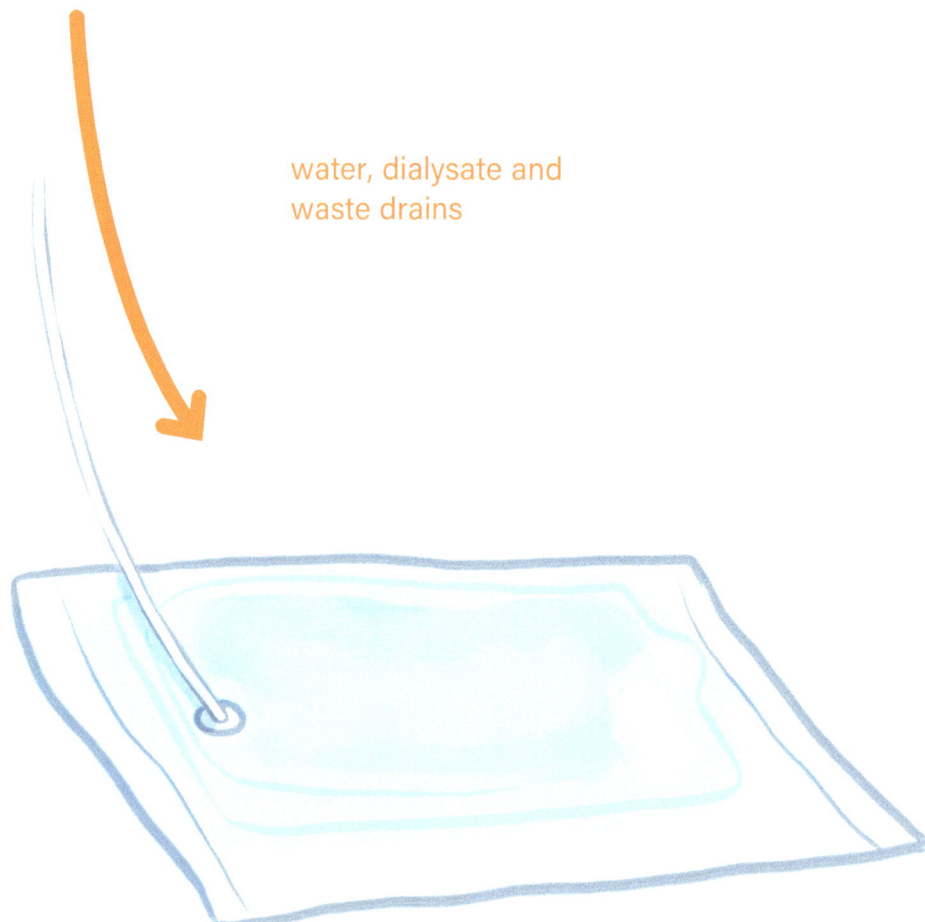

water, dialysate and waste drains

With PD, your catheter is your "lifeline." Taking good care of your catheter can prevent trips to the doctor and hospital.

To take the best care of your catheter:

DO THESE:

✔ **Always** wash your hands before handling your catheter.

✔ **Clean the skin** around your catheter daily. (Your nurse will teach you how to do this.)

✔ Perform your exchanges **in a clean place**, using the steps you were taught.

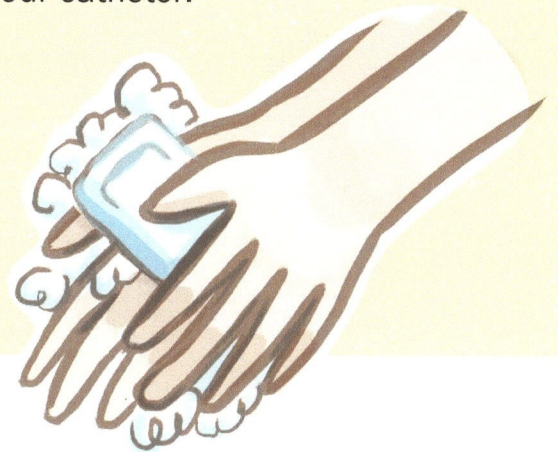

DO NOT:

✗ pull or tug at your catheter or wear clothes that rub it

✗ let your catheter flop around (Hold it in place as taught by your nurse.)

✗ damage your catheter

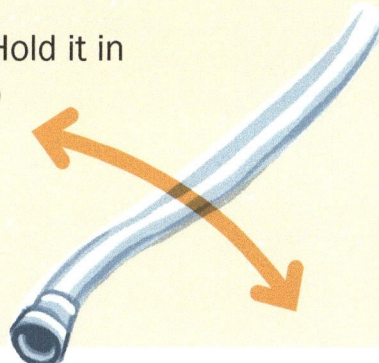

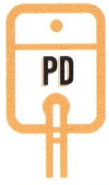

What problems can happen with PD?

Catheter infection, or "exit site" infection, can happen anytime germs get to your catheter. This is why you need to take good care of your catheter and the skin around it.

You may have an exit site infection if you notice any of these in the area around your catheter:

- tender to the touch

- red looking skin

- skin too warm

- drainage near the place your catheter enters your body

If you notice any of these, call your doctor's office at once. If not caught early and treated, an infection can cause you to lose your catheter. You may be able to get another catheter, or you may have to go on hemodialysis.

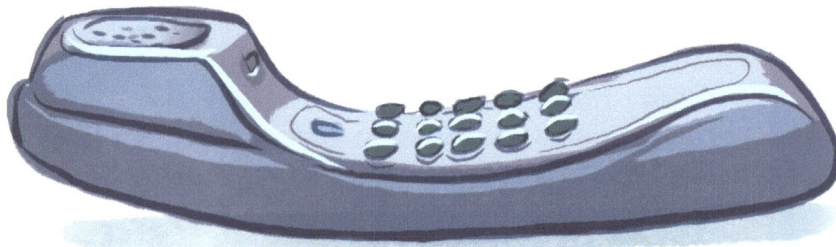

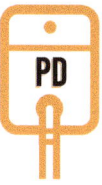

Infection inside the belly (peritonitis) may happen if you are on PD. It is caused when germs get inside your belly. This type of infection may be very painful and can be serious if not treated quickly.

You may have peritonitis if you have:

- pain that spreads through your belly and around your trunk

- fever, chills

- cloudy or bloody dialysate drained from your belly

- pieces of a stringy white substance in your drainage fluid

To treat this infection, your doctor will prescribe medicine (antibiotics) to mix with your dialysate. You may also need to take medicines by mouth or through your veins (IV's).

Take your medicine as often and for as many days as prescribed. This is true even if you feel you are well before you finish all the medicine. **If you don't take all of it, your infection can return or get much worse.**

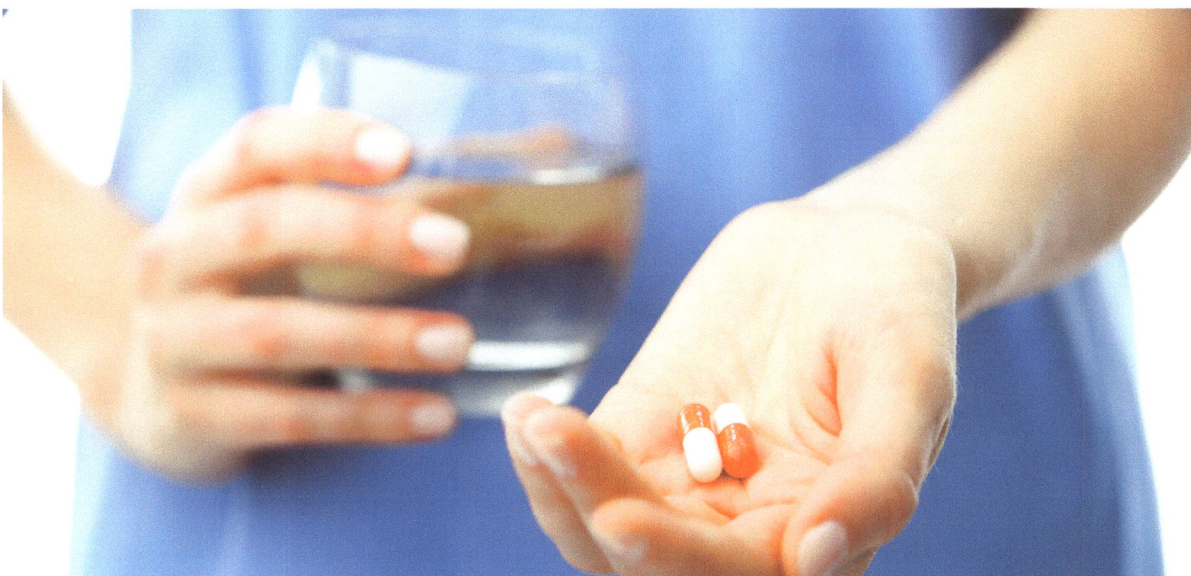

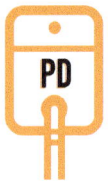

To **lower the risk** of getting peritonitis:

- Always follow all instructions given in your training program.

- Always check your dialysate bags. Never use a bag that leaks or has been punctured.

- Always clean your catheter and the place where the catheter attaches to the bag, as your nurse tells you.

- Never use cloudy dialysate.

- If you have cloudy drainage fluid, go see your doctor at once, and take the cloudy fluid with you.

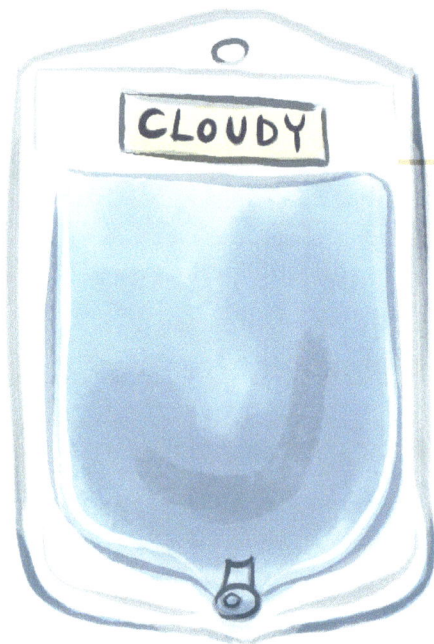

CLOUDY

Partly cloudy...
DON'T USE.

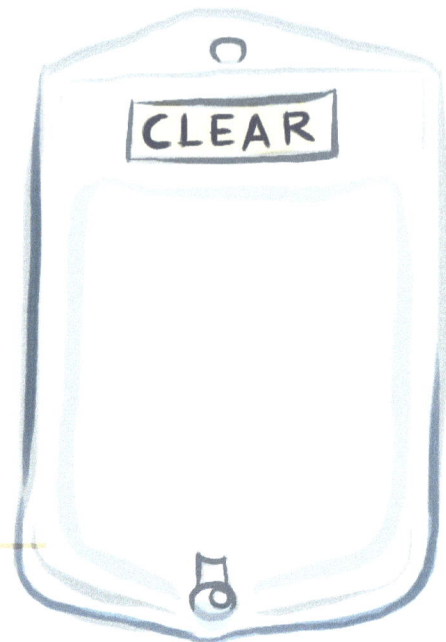

CLEAR

All clear...
OK to go!

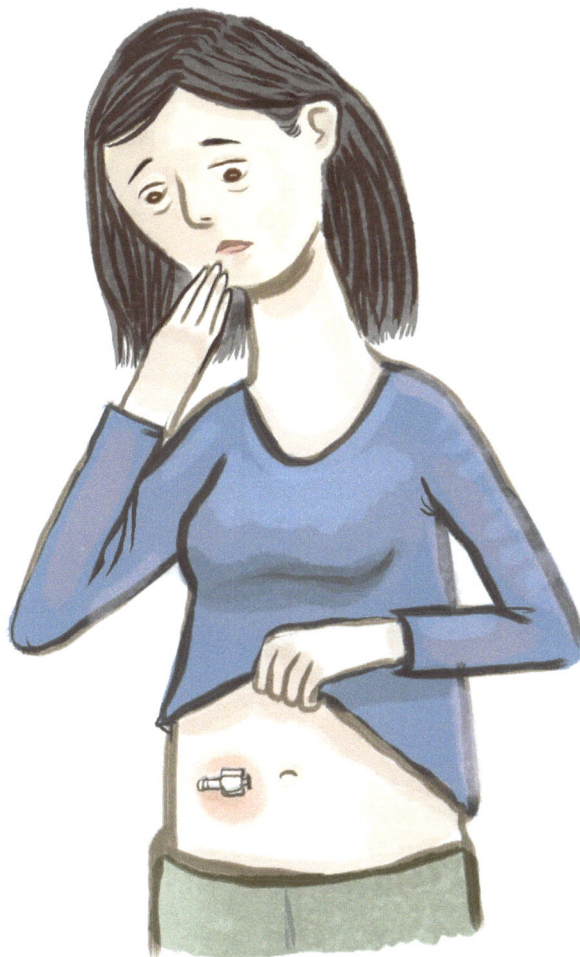

Other problems that may happen with PD and what to do about them:

- **pain when draining the fluid in or out**
  Make sure to warm your fluid before using, and let
  it in and out **slowly.**

- **tubing comes unhooked from catheter**
  Clamp off the tubing and catheter, and call
  your nurse or clinic.

- **bloody drainage fluid**
  You can have bloody drainage without an infection. But if
  this happens, tell your nurse or doctor right away.

- **trouble getting the fluid to go in or out of your belly**
  This can happen if you are constipated or have an infection.
  If this happens, call your doctor or nurse at once.

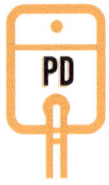

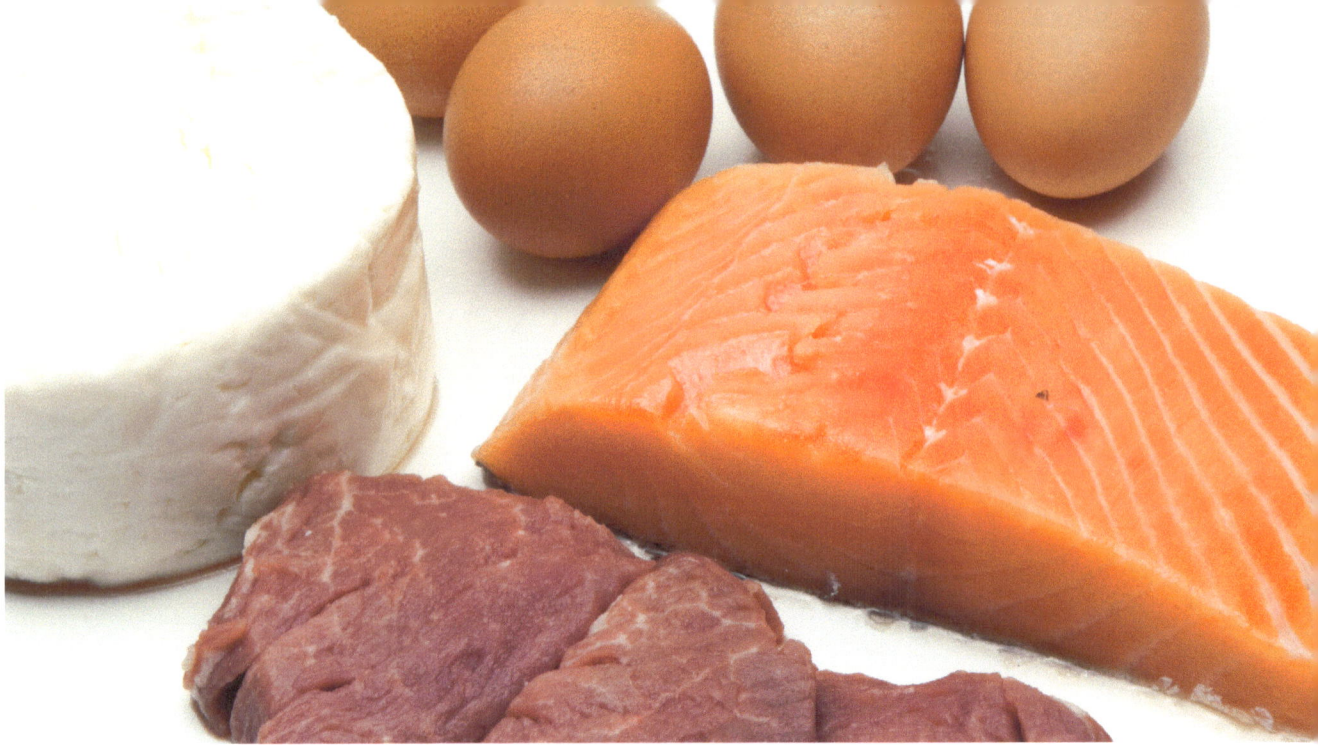

What to eat and drink while on PD?

With PD, your diet is decided by the results of your lab work.
Those on PD have fewer limits on their diet than those on hemo.

Protein

You will need to eat a high protein diet. This replaces the protein that is lost in the dialysis fluid. Foods that are high in protein are beef, pork, chicken, turkey, fish and eggs. You will need to eat plenty of them.

Potassium

When you're on PD, potassium is always being removed from your body. If tests show your potassium level is too high or low, your intake of potassium will need to be changed. **You may have to eat more or less of foods that are high in potassium** (most vegetables and fruits).

Phosphorus

You will have to limit the amount of phosphorus in your diet.
Phosphorus buildup in your blood makes you itch and leads to bone problems. These are some foods you will have to limit: milk and milk products, beans, nuts and dark colas.

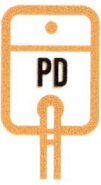

Fluid

You may have to limit the amount of fluid you drink. The amount of water removed from your body during PD treatments depends on the strength of your dialysis fluid. These foods are mostly fluid and will be limited: soft drinks, juice, ice, Jell-O, ice cream and puddings.

Sodium (salt)

You will need to limit the amount of sodium in your diet. These foods are high in sodium, so you can eat only small amounts of them: salt, soy sauce, pickles, chips, pretzels, lunch meats, hot dogs, cured meats (such as ham), canned foods, soups, most "quick" foods that come in a box and almost all fast foods.

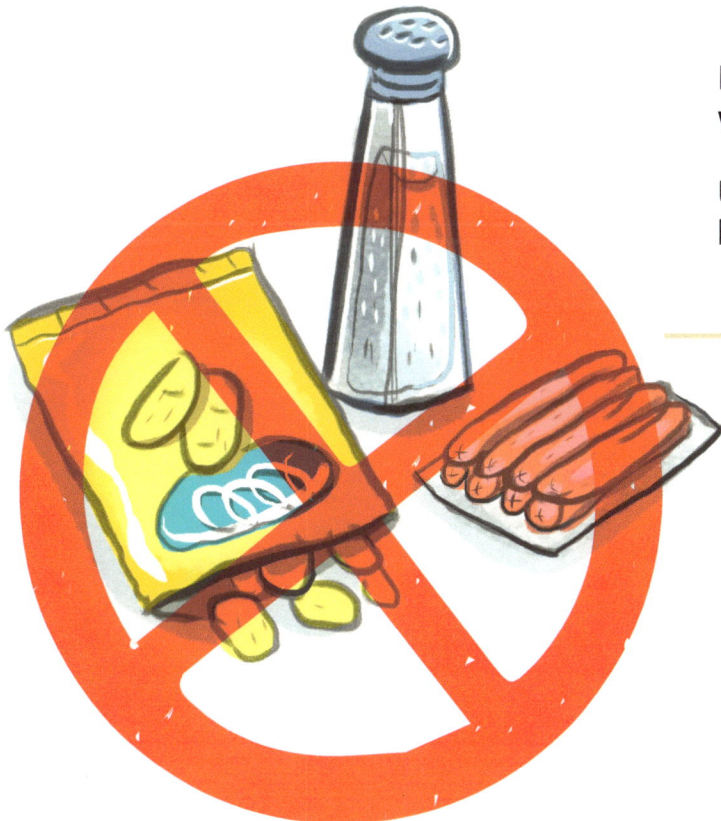

Learn how to keep a stable body weight by limiting fluids and salt.

Use the chart on page 47 to help keep up with your body weight.

More about hemo

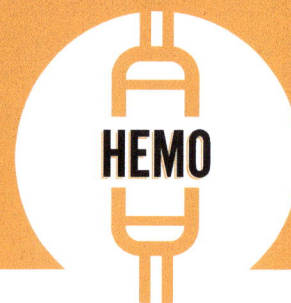

Hemo is most often done in a clinic, 3 times a week for 3 to 4 hours at a time. Some people do hemo at home. They and a helper must have a lot of special training, and a machine must be installed in the home.

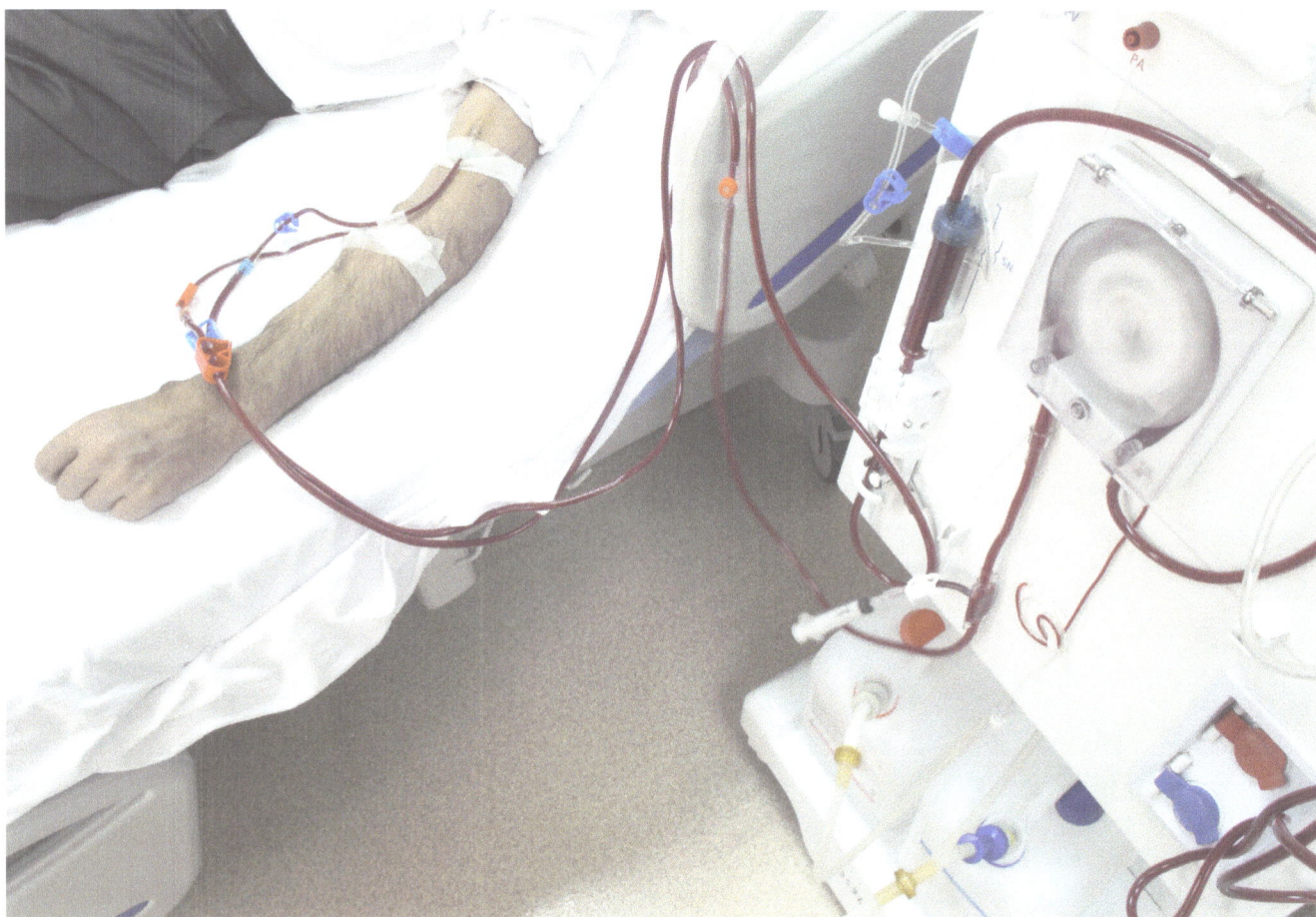

With hemo, an artificial kidney is used to clean your blood. The artificial kidney is placed on a machine which helps it do its work. Next, two needles are placed in your arm and hooked to plastic tubes. One tube takes a small amount of blood to the dialysis machine to be cleaned. The other tube returns the cleansed blood to your body.

During the treatment, very small amounts of blood are always going to the machine and coming back (returning) into your body. No more than about one cup of blood at a time is outside your body.

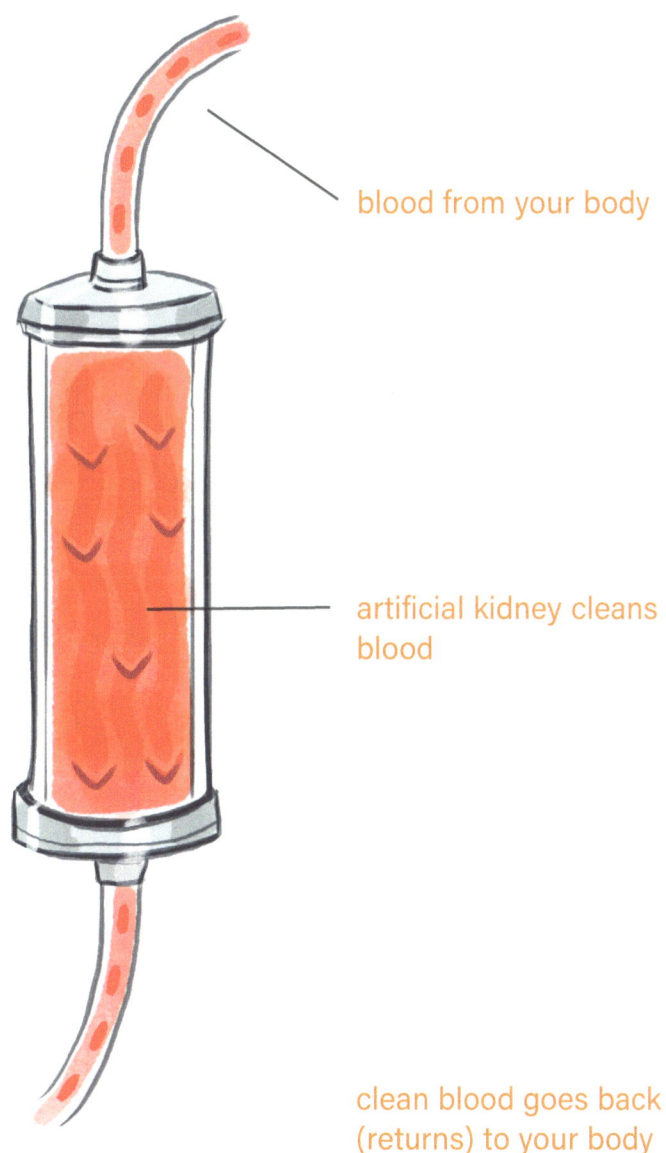

blood from your body

artificial kidney cleans blood

clean blood goes back (returns) to your body

You will need to have a way to get your blood into the artificial kidney each time you have a treatment. This is called an access, and it is most often put in your arm. To get your access, you will need a minor surgery that lasts about an hour. (Until you get this long-term access, you will have a tube for short-term access in your shoulder.)

One type of access is called a fistula, or A-V (arterial- venous) fistula. To make this, a doctor joins an artery and a vein under your skin.

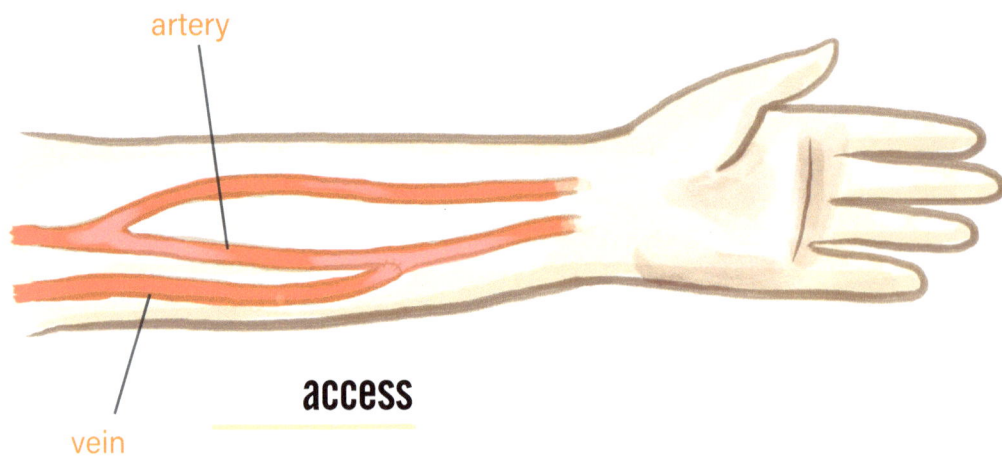

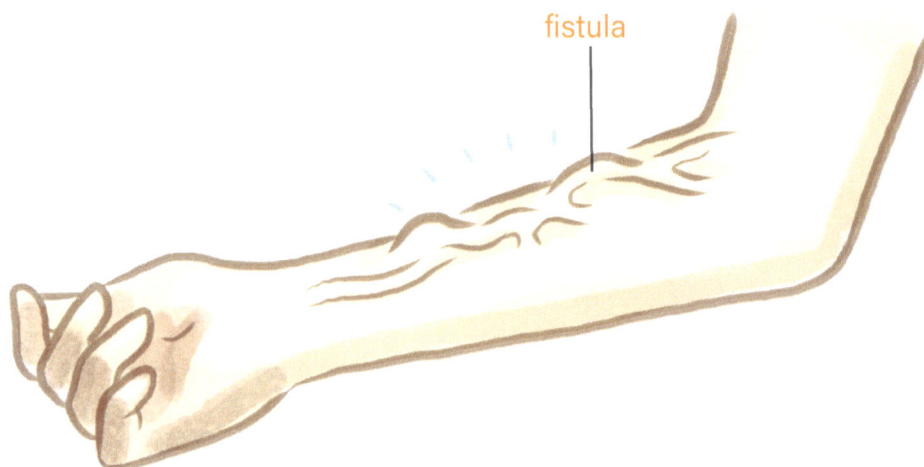

artery

access

vein

fistula

The other type of access is called a graft. A man-made tube is placed just under your skin. The surgeon sews one end to a vein and the other end to an artery.

Your access will cause a bump on your arm. If you touch it, you can feel the blood running through. (It is a vibrating feeling. Health workers call it a thrill or "buzz.") Grafts are most often ready to use in a few weeks. Fistulas may take up to a few months to be ready for use.

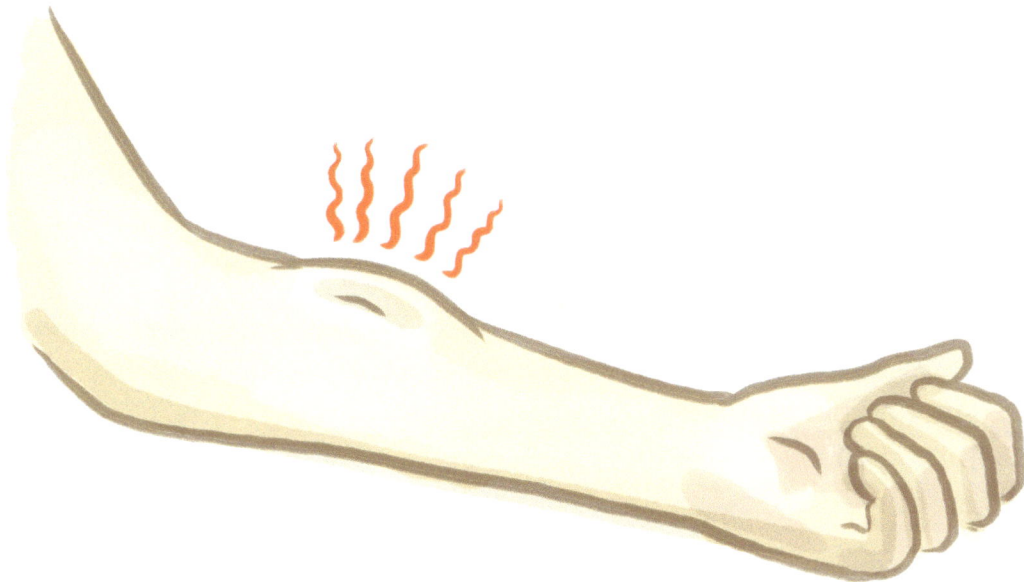

Having an access in an arm **does not** prevent you from using that arm. You must be careful about some things (see pages 32 and 33), but you can still do things like play tennis or go bowling.

Access care

With hemo, your access is your "lifeline," and it must have special care. The care is the same for a fistula or a graft. If your access is ruined by a clot, infection or for any other reason, you will have to go back to surgery and get another one. But there is a limit to the number of times this can be done.

These are some things you can do to keep your access in good shape:

▶ **No bleeding!**
Your access can bleed a lot if cut, so keep sharp objects away from it. If your access starts to bleed after a treatment, hold pressure on it, and call for help. Teach your family how to do this, too.

▶ **Always have a thrill!**
Make sure the blood is flowing by feeling for the buzz or thrill each morning, night and a few times during the day. This is the best way to know that your access still has blood flowing through it.

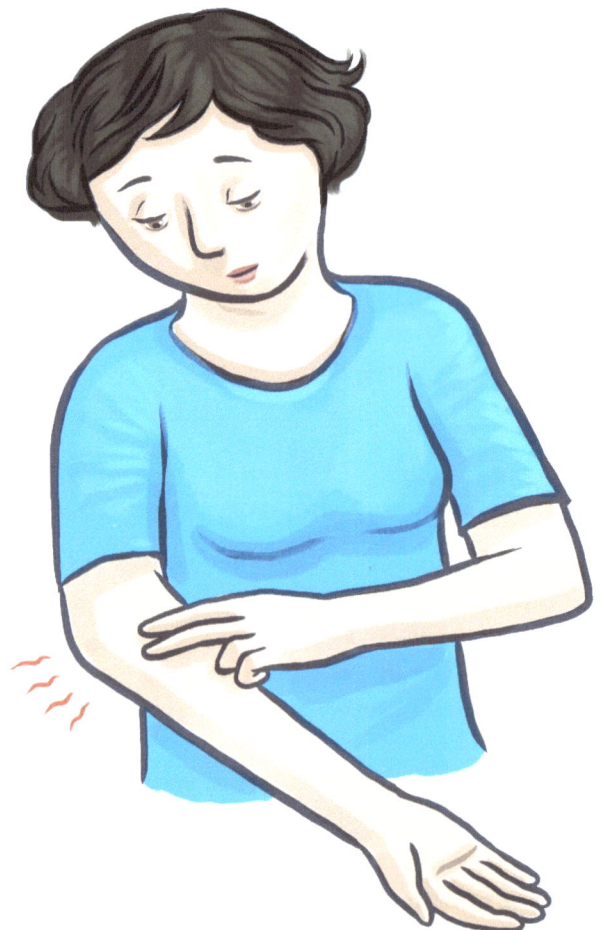

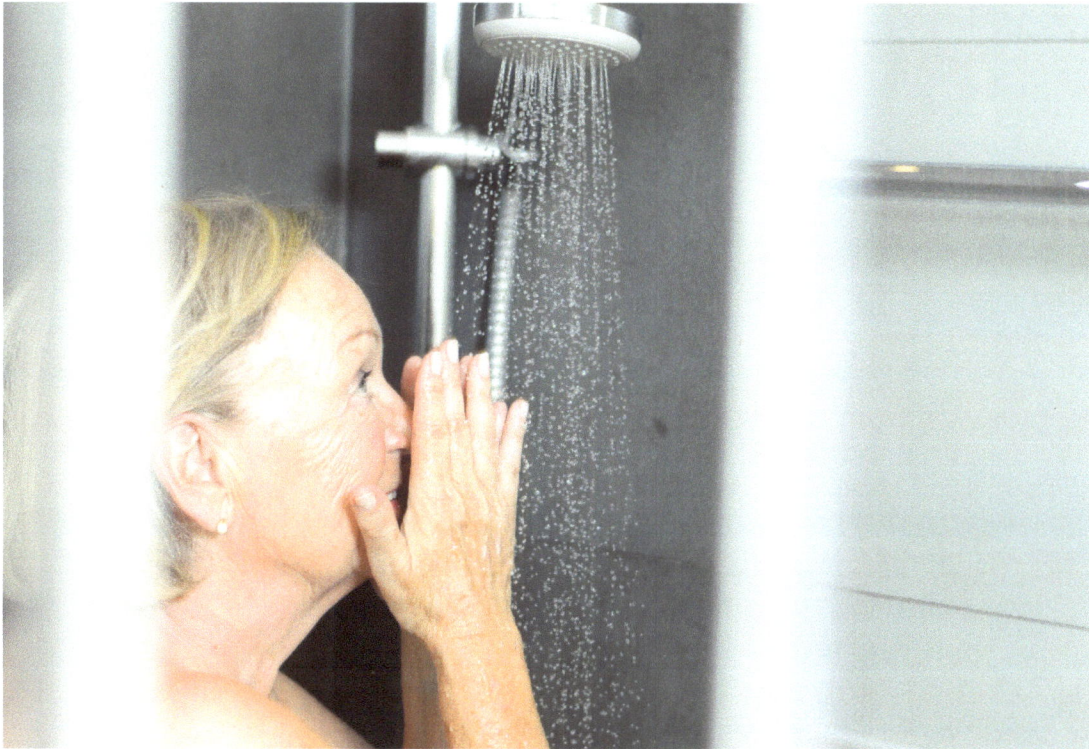

➡ Keep your access from clotting.

To prevent clots, don't wear tight clothes around your access or sleep on your access arm. Never let anyone take your blood pressure, draw blood or stick a needle in that arm (except for your treatment). If you think you may have a clot (you can't feel the "buzz"), call your doctor at once. He or she may be able to remove the clot if it is caught soon enough.

➡ Keep it clean.

The needles used for your treatments leave holes where infection can enter. To help prevent infection: Wash your hands often, and keep your body clean. Before a treatment, your nurse or technician will clean the skin over your access. After it is cleaned, do not touch this area, and don't touch it while the needle is in. After each treatment, a small bandage will be placed over the skin where the needles were. Leave this on until that night or the next day.

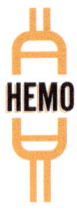

Problems that can happen during hemo

Call for help at once if you notice any of these:

- irregular heartbeat
- chest pain
- bleeding from access

If you have any of the problems listed below during a treatment, let your nurse know. Often there are ways to prevent or relieve these:

- fever and chills
- vomiting or feeling sick to your stomach
- shortness of breath
- muscle cramps
- feeling hot and flushed
- feeling lightheaded or dizzy
- headache

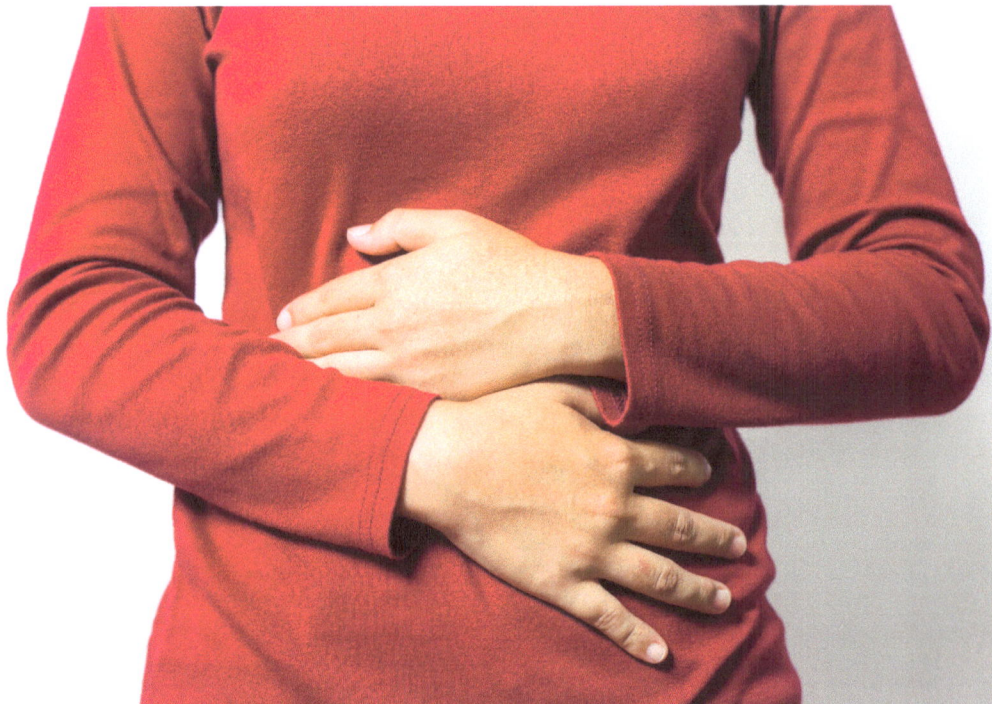

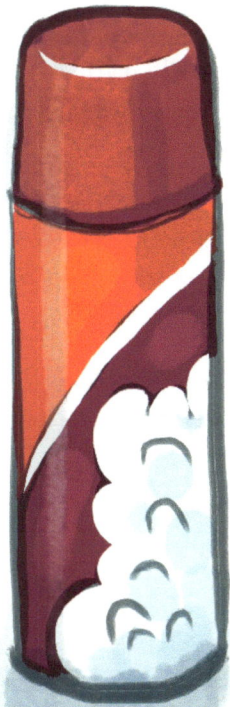

Wait 4 to 6 hours
before shaving

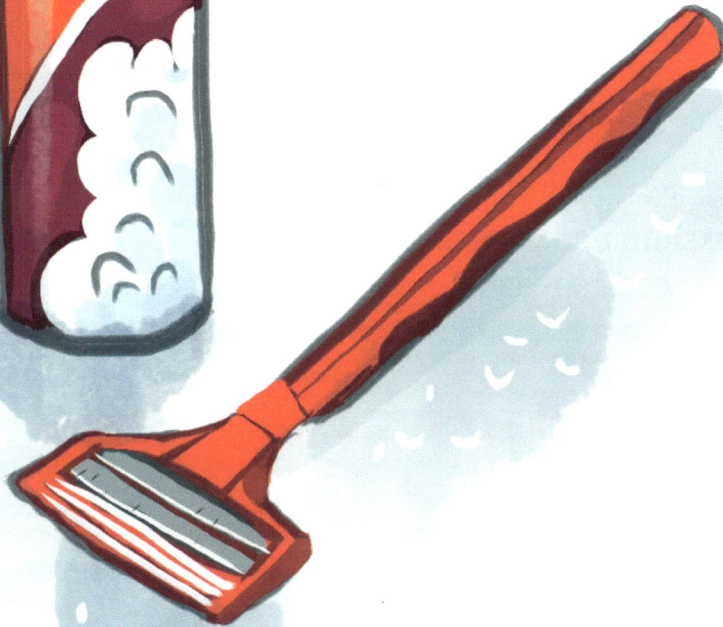

What about after treatment?

Before each treatment, you will get a blood thinner to keep the blood from clotting while it is in the artificial kidney. Your blood remains very thin for 4 to 6 hours after you "come off the machine." During this time, **don't** shave, work with saws or sharp objects like knives or needles, and **do** drive carefully.

What food and drink to limit while on hemo

With hemo, your blood is cleaned 3 times a week. Fluid and waste build up between treatments. To keep waste and fluid levels from getting too high, you must follow the diet you are given.

A dietitian will teach you about your diet and how to prepare your food. It will most likely not be what you are used to, and you may not enjoy your new food at first. But you need to eat well to stay healthy, so hang in there. Most people find they enjoy the new diet once they get used to the changes. Some of the changes you will need to make are discussed on the next pages.

The main things that change with your new diet are **fluids, sodium (salt), potassium** and **phosphorus.** You may also need to eat more **protein.** Your body needs about 8 ounces of good protein a day. Good proteins come from animal sources such as meats, dairy foods and fish.

Learn how to keep a stable body weight by limiting fluids and salt.

Use the chart on page 47 to help keep up with your body weight.

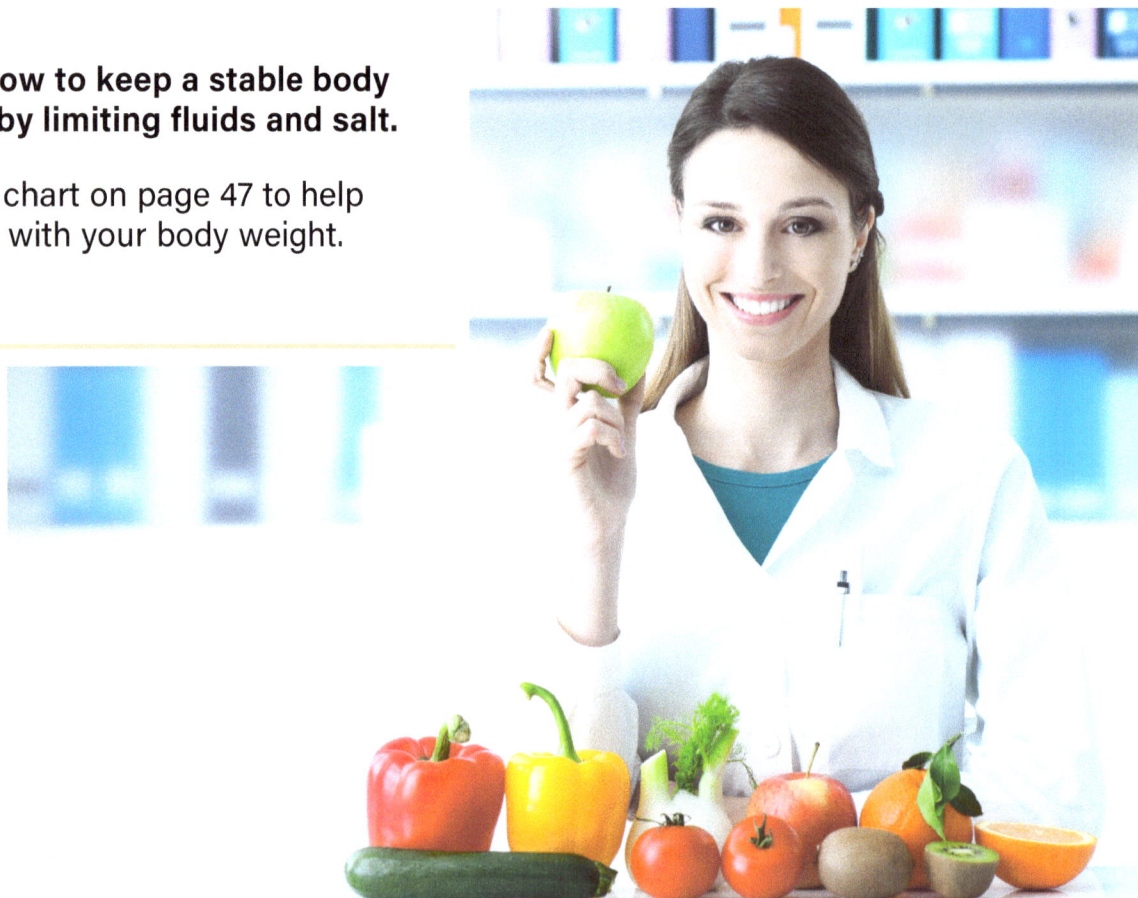

With hemo, you must limit **all** of these:

Fluid

Because your body can't get rid of it, you must limit the amount of fluid you take in. Signs of too much fluid are: swelling of feet, legs, ankles or face; shortness of breath; increase in blood pressure and quick weight gain. **All** fluids count toward your daily limit, as do all foods that contain a lot of fluid. These include: Jell-O, ice cream, puddings, ice.

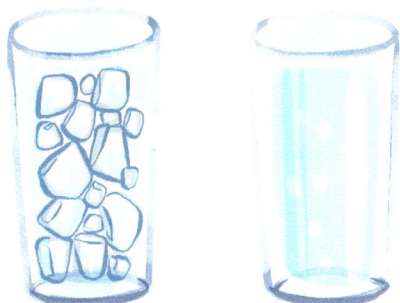

One full glass of ice equals ½ glass of water.

Sodium (salt)

Sodium buildup causes high blood pressure and heart failure. Signs of high sodium are swelling, thirst, dry mouth and dry tongue. Some foods that have a lot of sodium are: salt, pickles, chips, pretzels, lunch meats, hot dogs, cured meats (such as ham), canned foods, soups, most "quick" foods that come in a box and almost all fast foods.

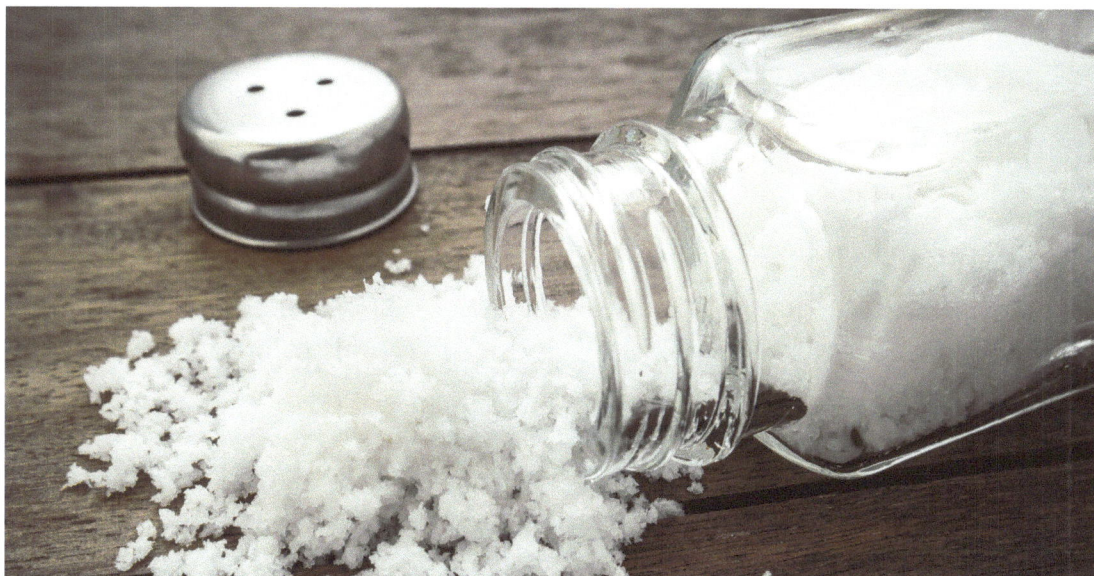

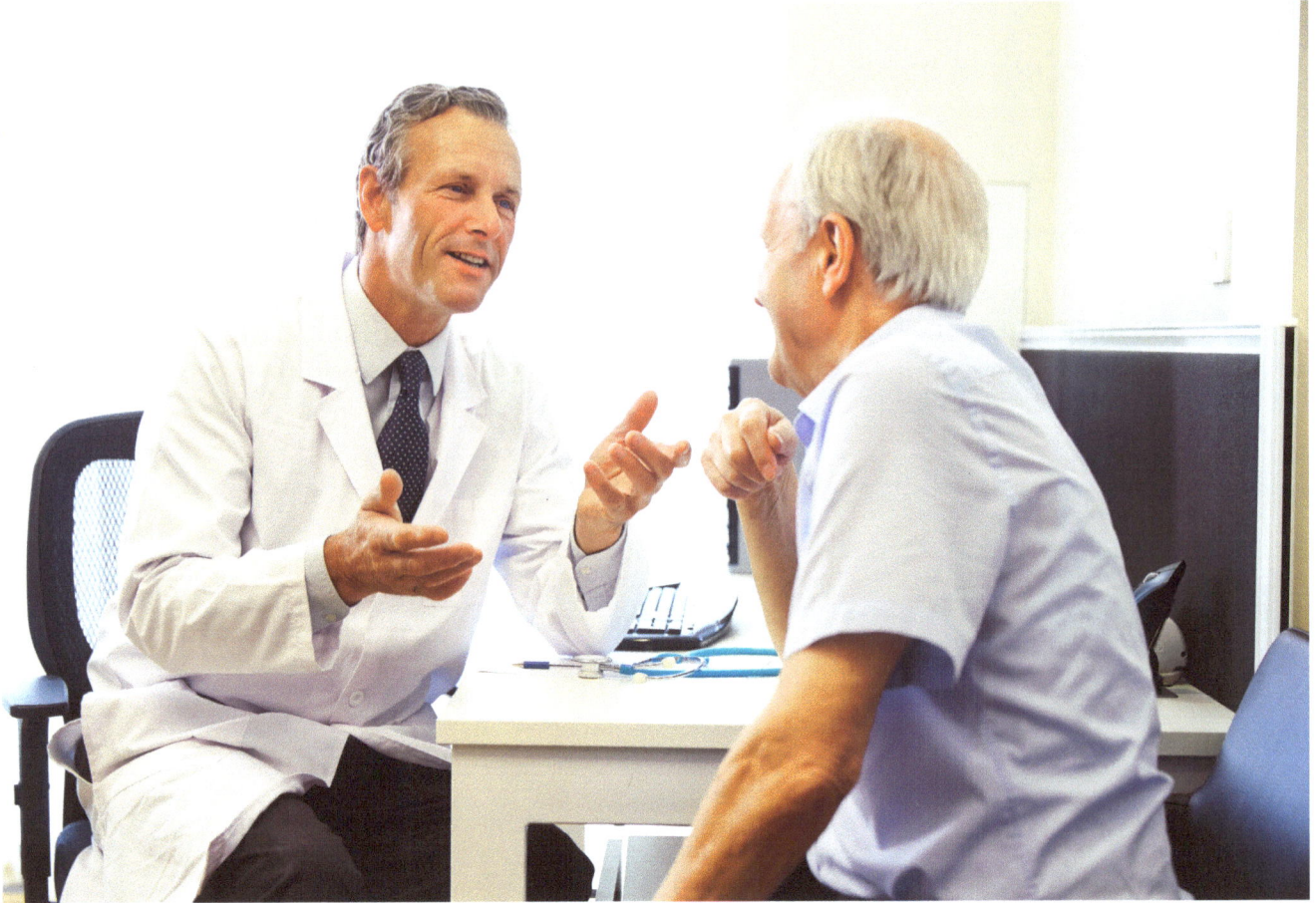

Potassium

If potassium builds up in your blood, it can cause **severe** heart problems. You may feel weak or have chest pain or skipped heartbeats. (If this happens, call your doctor at once.) Foods high in potassium include certain fruits and vegetables, nuts, beans, chocolate and salt substitute.

Phosphorus

Phosphorus buildup in your blood makes you itch and can lead to bone problems. Milk (and milk products such as ice cream, cheese, yogurt, etc.) are usually limited in this diet. Foods also high in phosphorus include beans, nuts and dark colas.

Your doctor and dietitian will decide what's right for you and will tell you the exact amounts of each food to eat. Your lab work will show how well your diet is working.

What you can eat

Here are some foods that may be OK for you to eat. Many of your favorites may be on the list. Look over this page, then talk to your doctor, nurse or dietitian to plan a few sample meals for yourself on the next pages.

Protein

Beef
Pork (chops or roast — not sausage)
Wild game
Chicken
Turkey
Fish
Eggs

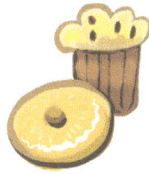

Starches

Bagels, muffins, english muffins
Yeast rolls, popovers
Bread (white, wheat, rye, pita)
Cornbread
Cereals (Cream of Wheat, grits, oatmeal: do not add salt, avoid instant cereals)
Crackers (unsalted)
Dry cereal (no nuts or dried fruit)
Noodles, rice
Pancakes, waffles
Popcorn
Tortillas (corn or flour)

Fruits

Apples, applesauce
Blueberries, cherries
Cranberry sauce
Fruit cocktail
Grapes
Lemons, limes, tangerines Pears, plums, pineapple Raspberries, strawberries

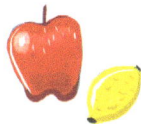

Vegetables

Beets
Cabbage
Carrots (cooked)
Celery, cucumbers
Cooked broccoli and cauliflower
Corn
Eggplant
Green beans, peas (sweet)
Lettuce
Onion
Pepper (green & red)
Squash (yellow), zucchini
Turnips, rutabagas

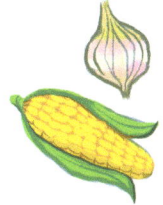

Fats

Butter, margarine
Cooking oil
Cream cheese
Mayonnaise
Nondairy creamer
Salad dressings

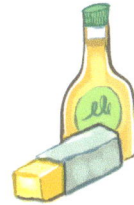

Sweets and Desserts

Cakes (pound, angel food, layer with icing)
Cookies (ginger snaps, lemon or vanilla filled, sugar, shortbread)
Cheesecake
Cinnamon rolls, doughnuts (glazed, jelly)
Fruit tarts
Pies (apple, blueberry, cherry, lemon, strawberry)
Popsicles
Rice Krispie treats
Honey, jam, jelly, syrup

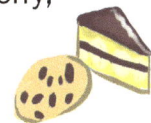

Beverages

Gingerale, Sprite, 7-Up
KoolAid, lemonade
Weak coffee & tea

If you have diabetes, be sure to talk to your health care provider for meal planning.

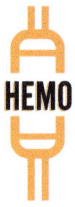

Sample menus

Here are sample menus planned from the list of foods you can eat. Try using the blank space to plan some meals for yourself. Serving sizes vary based on your calorie and protein needs. Ask your dietition what's right for you.

	Day 1	Day 2	Day 3
	Breakfast	**Breakfast**	**Breakfast**
Protein:	an egg	Canadian bacon	
Starch:	bagel	cinnamon toast	
Fruit:	fresh strawberries	applesauce	
Fat:	cream cheese	margarine	
Beverage:	coffee or tea	coffee or tea	
Milk:	milk	yogurt	
	Lunch	**Lunch**	**Lunch**
	Pasta salad made of:		
Protein:	canned tuna (no salt)	hamburger	
Vegetable:	sweet peas	lettuce	
Vegetable:	red pepper		
Starch:	pasta	hamburger bun	
Fat:	Italian dressing (no salt)	mayonnaise	
Fruit:	canned peaches	tangerine	
Dessert:	gingersnaps	Rice Krispie treat	
Beverage:	lemonade	coffee or tea	
	Dinner	**Dinner**	**Dinner**
Protein:	grilled fish	fried chicken	
Vegetable:	fresh asparagus	green beans	
Vegetable:	corn on the cob	yellow squash	
Starch:	yeast rolls	cornbread	
Fat:	margarine	margarine	
Fruit:	cheesecake	pound cake	
Dessert:	blueberry topping	strawberries	
Beverage:	coffee or tea	iced tea	

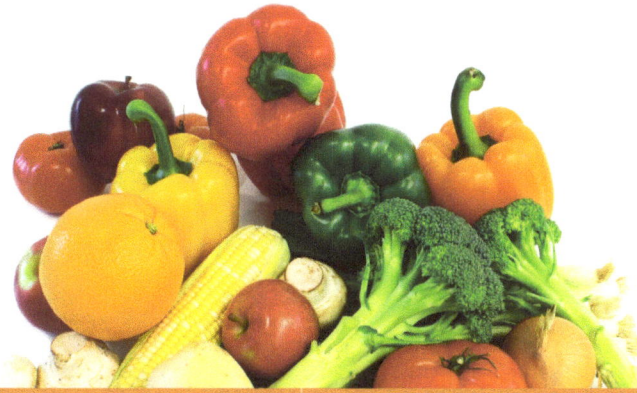

	Day 4	Day 5	Day 6
	Breakfast	**Breakfast**	**Breakfast**
Protein:			
Starch:			
Fruit:			
Fat:			
Beverage:			
Milk:			
	Lunch	**Lunch**	**Lunch**
Protein:			
Vegetable:			
Vegetable:			
Starch:			
Fat:			
Fruit:			
Dessert:			
Beverage:			
	Dinner	**Dinner**	**Dinner**
Protein:			
Vegetable:			
Vegetable:			
Starch:			
Fat:			
Fruit:			
Dessert:			
Beverage:			

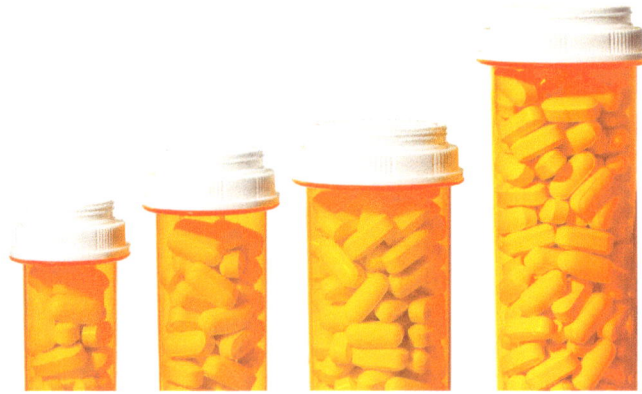

People on dialysis may take many medicines

Some medicines help get rid of waste products, and some replace things that are removed from your blood during treatments. Others are to control blood pressure or prevent the need for a blood transfusion.

Phosphate binders

Phosphate is contained in almost all foods. Milk and milk products (ice cream, cheese, yogurt) are very high in phosphate. When your kidneys are healthy, they get rid of the phosphate from your foods, but with kidney failure, you must have another way to get rid of it. Medicines called phosphate binders latch onto the phosphates and carry them out through your bowels.

Calcium

Calcium and phosphate are closely related in the body. If your phosphate is high, your calcium is most often low. Having too little calcium can cause your bones to be weak and prone to break. Your doctor may prescribe a calcium supplement for you.

Vitamins

You need vitamins to feel good and for many body functions. During treatments, some vitamins are removed along with extra fluid. These are replaced by taking vitamin pills after each treatment and on the days between treatments.

Erythropoietin (epo)

This substance, made by the kidneys, helps your body make red blood cells. With kidney failure, you sometimes don't make enough epo, and your red blood cell count can get very low (anemia). This makes you feel weak and tired. Severe anemia can make you short of breath and can even cause death. (Severe problems can happen if your blood pressure is high and you take epo. So if you are on blood pressure medicine, be sure to take it as prescribed.)

Iron

Your body can't use epo to make red blood cells unless you also have enough iron. So you may also need to take iron pills or have iron given to you in your dialysis treatments.

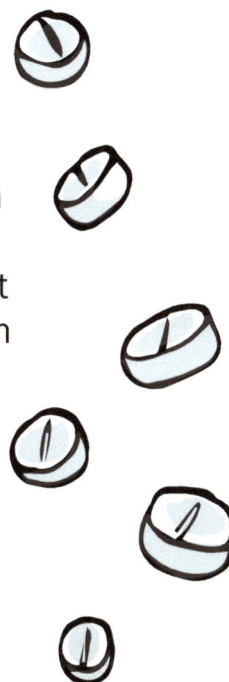

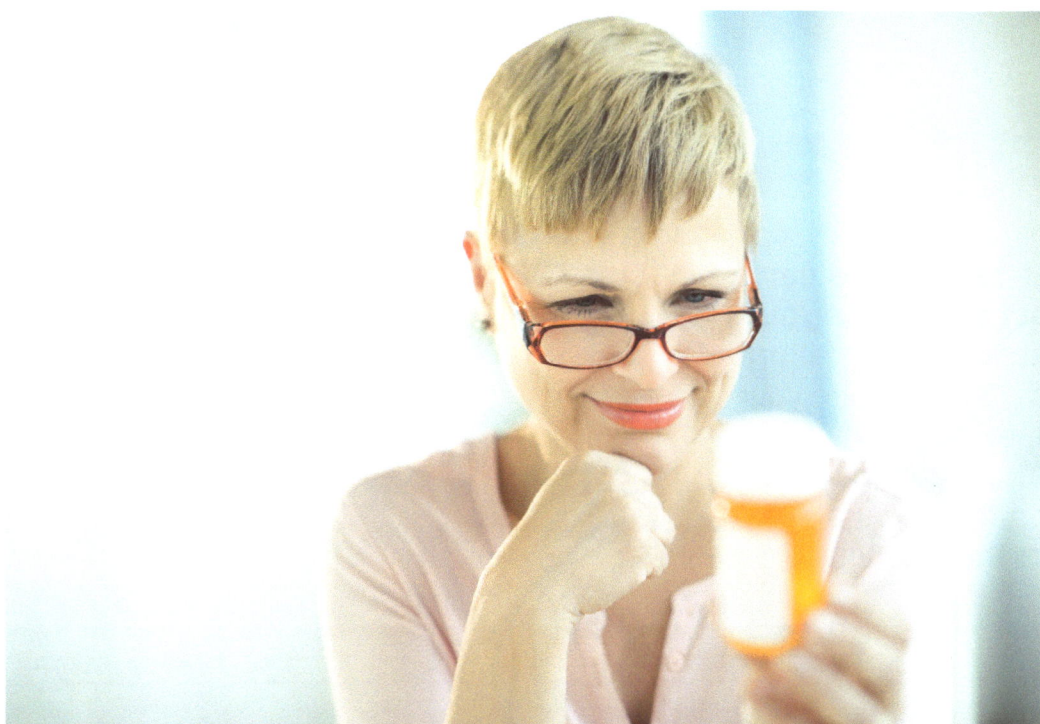

Blood pressure medicine

Many people with kidney failure also have high blood pressure. Your doctor may prescribe one or more medicines to control it. It is very important that you take these just as ordered. Check with your doctor to see if you should take your blood pressure medicine before your treatments.

On page 48 is a chart to help you keep up with your medicines. You may want to photocopy the page and write on the copy. That way, you can carry it in your purse or wallet, and if your medicines change, you can make a new copy and fill it out.

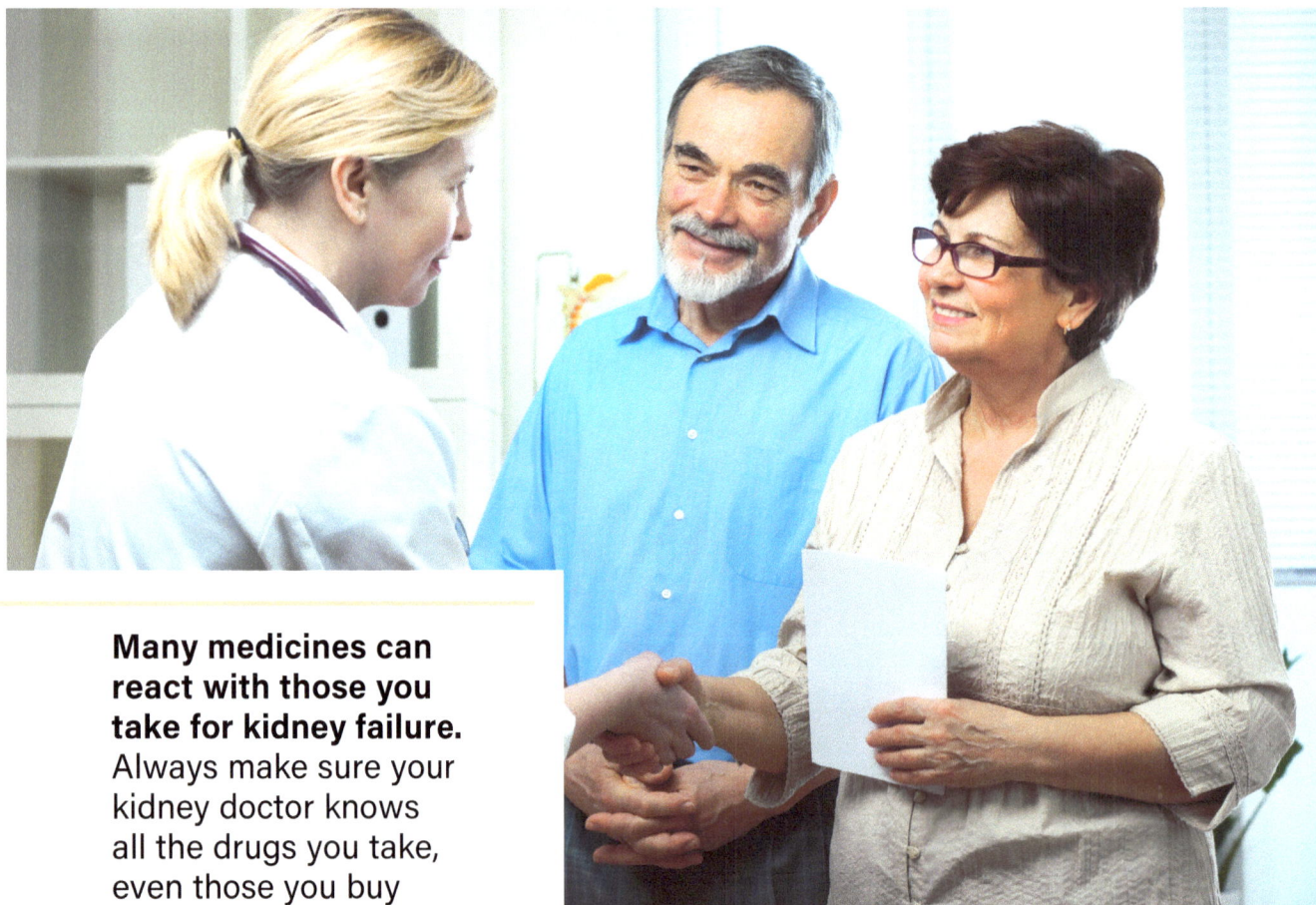

Many medicines can react with those you take for kidney failure. Always make sure your kidney doctor knows all the drugs you take, even those you buy over the counter.

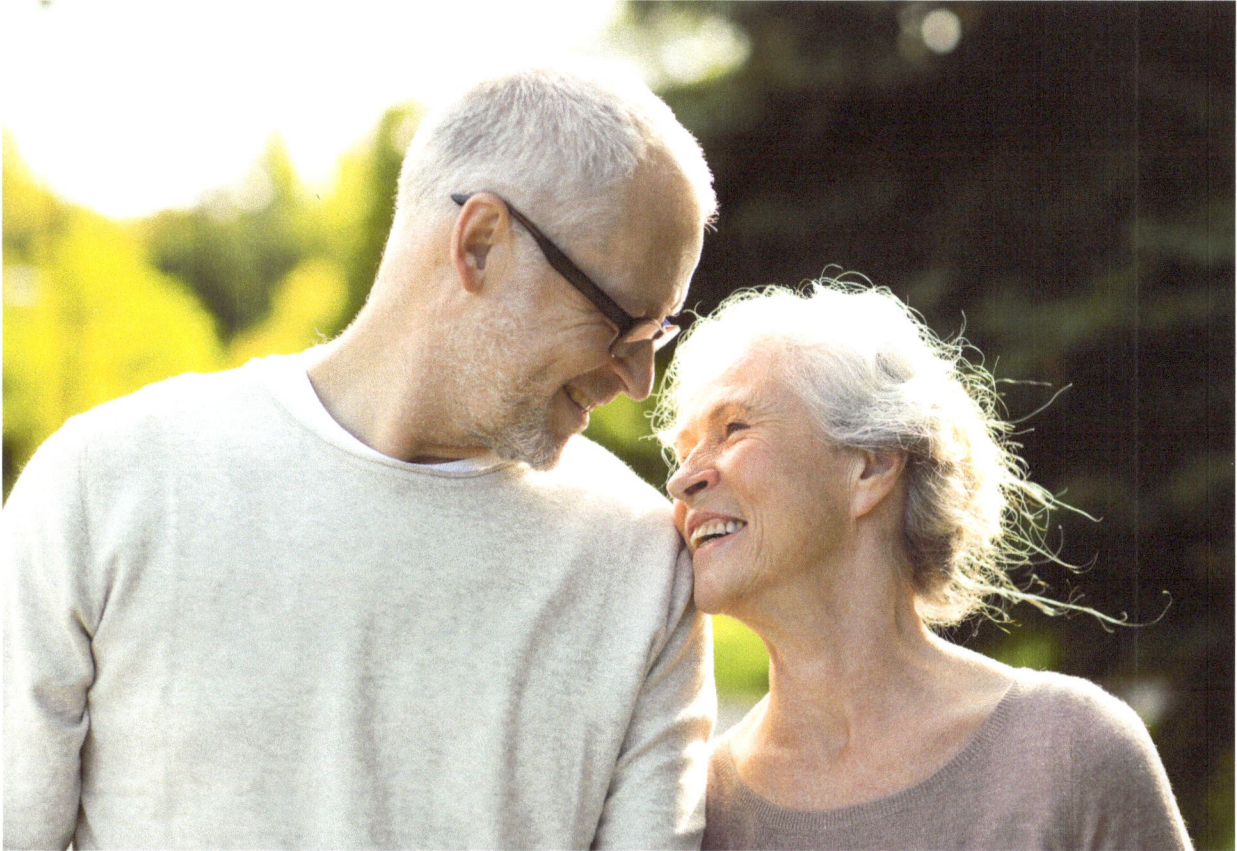

What's ahead

No matter how you look at it, living with kidney failure is tough. But you can learn to have a good life, even with the changes that kidney failure brings. Use all the help you can to get started with your new life. Call on your support team (page 10), write or call for help from the resources listed on page 46, and talk to friends, family and your health care team. Use the worksheets in this book to help plan meals and keep up with your medicines and changes in your body weight.

Please keep this book and read it several times (share it with your family too). Make a list of questions for your health care team and ask questions at your next appointment.

This book was written to help you understand kidney failure. Those who have it face many changes in their daily lives. We hope this book helped you understand these changes, as well as know about the different ways kidney failure is treated.

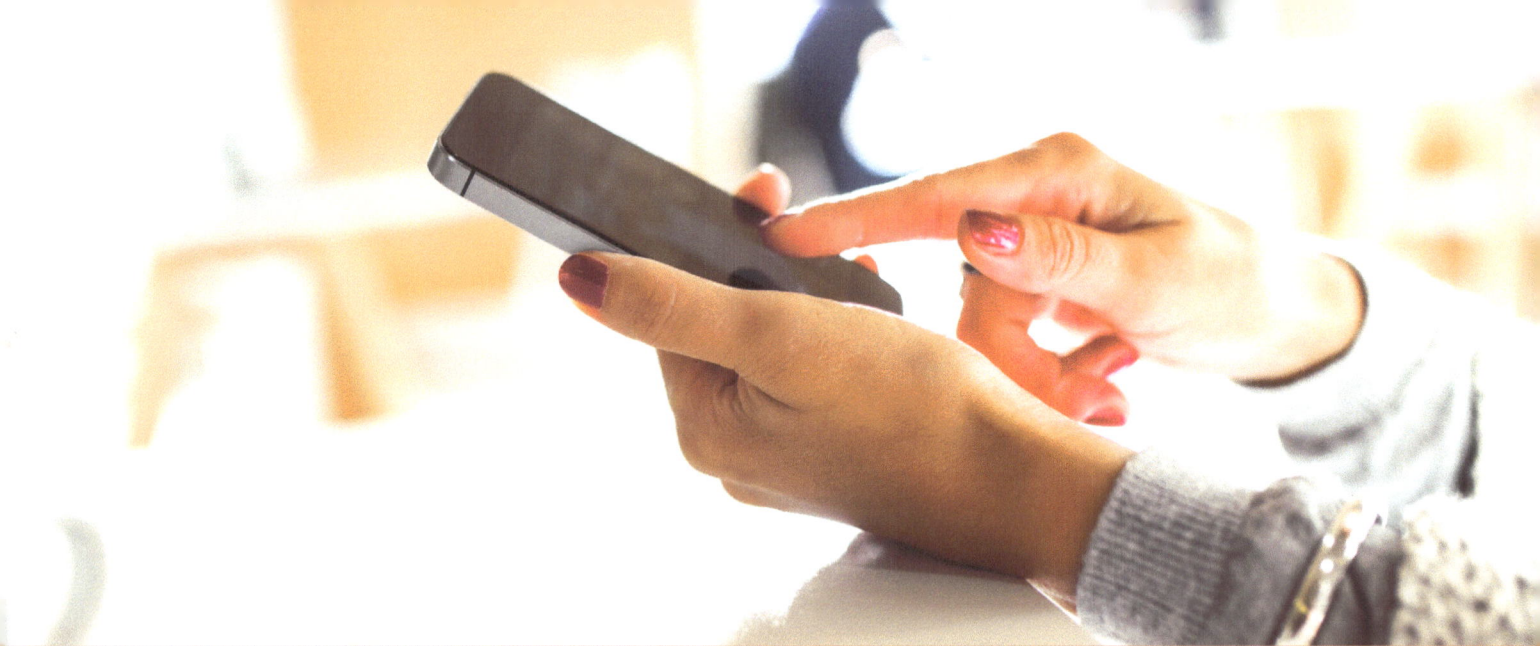

Resources

American Kidney Fund
11921 Rockville Pike, Ste. 300
Rockville, MD 20852
(800) 638-8299
kidneyfund.org

The National Kidney Foundation, Inc. (NKF)
30 East 33rd Street
New York, NY 10016
(800) 622-9010
kidney.org

Agency for Health Care Research and Quality
Office of Commuication and Knowledge Transfer
5600 Fishers Lane, 7th Floor
Rockville, MD 20857
(301) 427-1104
ahrq.gov

American Association of Kidney Patients (AAKP)
14440 Bruce B. Downs Blvd.
Tampa, FL 33613
(800) 749-2257
aakp.org

Weight chart

Use this chart daily to keep track of your body weight.

My normal body weight range is:

_____

(Ask your doctor or nurse to tell you these numbers.)

date	weight	date	weight

Medicine chart

Doctor:_____

address_____

_____

phone_____

Pharmacy:

address_____

_____

phone_____

Dialysis Clinic:

address_____

_____

phone_____

drug name	purpose	when to take	how much	things to watch for